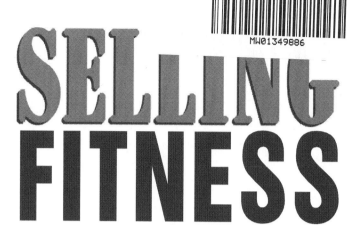

Free online sales training

We now offer a series of free sales training videos on the Internet. You can access the videos and weekly sales tips at www.HealthClubSalesTraining.com

Sell more memberships with professional training!

Your salespeople can probably sell more memberships; they just need the proper training and development. It costs thousands to have Casey Conrad comeand deliver her two-day Sales Boot Camp at your club and your entire membership staff is off the floor during that time. Give every new and existing salesperson this entire sales training course online! To obtain more information go to: www.caseyconrad.com/aboutSFP

Contact Casey Conrad

If you have any questions or would like to contact Casey you can do so at:
Casey@CaseyConrad.com
401-792-7009

What others are saying about Selling Fitness

Selling Fitness is a great contribution to the fitness industry. It gives you a comprehensive guide to sales strategies and systems that are proven effective for maximizing membership sales.
    James E. Smith, President
    Peak Performance International Fitness Network

Selling Fitness can save clubs years of trial and error sales training. We recently spent months designing and scripting our sales process. This book would have saved untold hours and dollars. A must for every club interested in improving sales.
    Mark Eisenzimmer
    Owner/General Manager, Cascade Athletic Club

An absolute must read for every membership staff person in the industry. There are many sound, basic philosophies and new ideas throughout the book. Selling Fitness is a very interesting, informative, and well written book.
    Ray Gordon
    Salesmakers

This book is a must read for anyone who is selling health club memberships or is about to start selling memberships. It can only help you sell more.
    Bruce Carter
    President, Optimal Fitness Systems Int'l.

A concise and comprehensive guide to selling health and fitness memberships. This book is informative, entertaining, and easy reading. Conrad's approach to selling is an invaluable bridge between the dream world of ideas and the real world of sales. The examples alone are worth thier weight in gold. A must read for those involved in the industry.

    Frank Bingham, Jr., Ed.D, Ph.D.
    Professor of Marketing, Bryant University

+Copyright 1994, 1995, 1996, 1999, 2008 by Casey Conrad
All Rights Reserved.

Where noted, there are certain scripts and forms throughout this book that the author has intended the reader to copy or paraphrase for personal use at their job as a salesperson.

No other part of this book may be reproduced or transmitted in any form or by any means, electronic, mechanical, including photocopying, recording, or by any information storage and retrieval system, except in the case of reviews, without the express written permission of the publisher, except where permitted by law.

Published by: Communication Consultants, WBS, Inc.
                     11 Kenyon Avenue
                     Wakefield, RI 02879
                     401-792-7009
                     401-783-9671 (fax)
                     Commcon@verizon.net

Illustrations by: Jeff Bursette
                     57 Frookdale Street
                     Cumberland, RI 02864
                     401-333-1798

ACKNOWLEDGMENTS

First, I want to thank my mother, Carol H. Conrad, and my father, Robert L. Conrad, for their support. Each instilled in me the desire to be the best I can and the tenacity to finish what I start.

Next I want to thank the rest of my family and all of my friends. I could not have asked for a better "editorial support team." You listened at all hours of the day and night, laughed when I needed it most, and kept me motivated throughout the writing of this book. For this, many, many thanks!

In memory of Rob

His Unconditional love.
His incredible courage.
His big, bright smile.
His contagious laugh.
His Thunder.

Icons Used in this Book

To alert you to special passages of text that you especially may want to read or pay attention to, icons have been placed in the margins to help guide you. Below is a description of what each icon means:

 "Key Point."

 "Hot Tip."

 "Core Skill."

 "Good Idea."

Table of Contents

INTRODUCTION 9

1. WHAT MOTIVATES PEOPLE TO BUY? 11
    - THE FORCES WITHIN YOU 12
    - USING THE FORCES IN SELLING 16
    - DISSATISFACTION LEADS TO ACTION 18

2. WHAT DO PEOPLE BUY? 23
    - PEOPLE BUY WANTS 24
    - THE CHALLENGE 25
    - WANTS ARE AN INDIVIDUAL THING 27
    - CONFLICTING WANTS 27

3. WHY BUY FROM YOU? 31
    - AN ATTITUDE ADJUSTMENT 31
    - EXCEED EXPECTATIONS 32
    - STAYING POWER 33
    - ANCHORING 33

4. RAPPORT & COMMUNICATION STYLES 39
    - WHAT IS RAPPORT? 40
    - COMMUNICATION STYLES 41
    - SPOTTING THE VISUAL COMMUNICATOR 41
    - HEARING THE AUDITORY COMMUNICATOR 45
    - GRASPING THE KINESTHETIC 48
    - AUDITORY DIGITAL 52
    - KEEPING THINGS IN PERSPECTIVE 52

5. ESTABLISHING RAPPORT 57
    - THE ELEMENTS OF COMMUNICATION 58
    - MATCHING AND MIRRORING 61
    - BODY POSTURE 63
    - MUSCULAR TENSION 64
    - FACIAL EXPRESSIONS 65
    - BREATHING 66
    - INTENT IS EVERYTHING 66
    - VOICE QUALITIES 67
    - APPLY YOUR NEW SKILLS 68

6. MAKING THE TELEPHONE WORK FOR YOU 71
- USE YOUR SKILLS 71
- THE INFORMATION CALL 73
- INFO CALL SCRIPT 74
- UNDERSTANDING THE INFO CALL 76
  - INTRODUCTION 76
  - PRE-QUALIFY 77
  - INFORMATION GATHERING 79
  - CLOSING 80
  - WRAP-UP 81
- TIME WELL SPENT 82
- EXCEPTION TO THE RULE 83
- WHY THE OBJECTIONS? 84
- BUT I JUST WANT THE PRICES! 85
- THE HOSTILE CALLER 87
- THE REALLY HOSTILE CALLER 90
- THE NON-COMMITTAL CALLER 91
- NEVER HANG UP EMPTY HANDED! 92
- BUILD A DATA BASE 93
- CONFIRMING APPOINTMENTS 95
- CALL-BACKS 97

7. THE PERSONAL ANALYSIS 105
- THE GREETING 105
- A NECESSARY ALTERNATIVE? 106
- GREETING WALK-INS 107
- GIVING THE BRIEF OVERVIEW 109
- THE ART OF PREFRAMING 110
- PREFRAMING THE PERSONAL ANALYSIS 111
- USING A PERSONAL ANALYSIS FORM 113
- EXERCISE HISTORY 114
  - THE EXERCISER 114
  - THE PREVIOUS EXERCISER 115
  - THE NON-EXERCISER 116
- GOALS AND MOTIVATION 117
- HEALTH HISTORY 120
- AVOID THE PITFALL 120
- SAMPLE PERSONAL ANALYSIS 122

8. THE TOUR 125
- THE TOUR ROUTE 125
- MOVE AT HIS PACE 127
- USING A FEATURE-BENEFIT-FEEDBACK SYSTEM 128
- TOO MUCH OF A GOOD THING? 130
- PREFRAME COMMON OBJECTIONS 131
- INTERACTIVE INFORMATION 133
- PRICE DROPPING 134
- MORE DIRECT TEST CLOSES 136

9. CLOSING & OVERCOMING OBJECTIONS 143
- A FINAL QUESTION 143
- PRESENT ALL MEMBERSHIPS 144
- PRESENT IN STAGES 144
- SHUT-UP! 146
- ASK FOR THE SALE 147
- WELCOME OBJECTIONS 148
- WHY OBJECTIONS? 148
- RELAX AND FEED IT BACK 150
- ALIGN WITH HIM 150
- QUESTION IT 151
- ISOLATE THE OBJECTION 151
- REFRAME 152
- CLOSE AGAIN 152
- ESTABLISH A COURSE OF CONTACT 154
- COMMON OBJECTIONS 155
  - I NEED TO THINK ABOUT IT 155
  - IT'S TOO EXPENSIVE 156
  - I WANT TO CHECK OUT OTHER CLUBS 158
  - I'M NOT SURE I AM GOING TO
  - STICK WITH IT 160
  - I NEED TO TALK TO MY SPOUSE 161

10. THE POWER OF PROSPECTING 165
- STRENGTH IN NUMBERS 166
- TAKING THE RESPONSIBILITY 167
- CAST YOUR NETS! 168
- THE BEST KEPT SECRET 168
- HAVING THE PASSES 169
- THE FORMAT 170
- BUDDY REFFERAL FORM 172
- WHEN TO BR? 172
- THE PRESENTATION 174
- DEALING WITH OBJECTIONS 175
- WHEN TO CONTACT NEW BR'S 178
- THE BR CALL 178
- SHOULD I CLOSE? 180
- EXISTING MEMBER REFERRALS 180
- TRACKING EXISTING MEMBER BR'S 181
- GUEST PASS TRACKING FORM 182
- CREATIVELY GENERATING LEADS 183
- PERSONAL PROSPECTING 183
- PROMOTIONAL PROSPECTING 186

11. LEAD MANAGEMENT **193**
    WHY LEAD MANAGEMENT? 193
    THE CHALLENGE 195
    SETTING UP THE SYSTEM 197
    IT'S EASY TO USE! 197
    ENHANCING THE SYSTEM 199
    DO IT NOW! 199
    KEEP ACCURATE NOTES 200

CONCLUSION **205**

INTRODUCTION

Remember Jack Lalanne? He was that lean, agile man who made himself known to thousands of Americans in the 1960's appearing on their black and white television sets with a daily program of exercise and calisthenics. I can vividly remember my grandmother eagerly following this man who wore a tight blue-green jumpsuit, doing jumping jacks, deep knee bends, sit-ups and a host of other exercises. Jack Lalanne was to the 60's what Richard Simmons and Jane Fonda were to the 80's and "Body By Jake" is to the 90's. Currently, Lalanne has a chain of health clubs he franchises and can be seen on cable television-in his 70's- doing one-arm push-ups, pull-ups and full splits while promoting a juice machine. Even with all his optimism, I doubt Jack Lalanne would foresee that by 2007, there would be 29,636 commercial health clubs in the US, that 44.1 million Americans would be members of those clubs and that the industry would reach 18.5 billion dollars in revenue.*

Today, the health and fitness industry continues to change and evolve as it has in the past. In the 1970's racquetball clubs and women's figure salons were in demand. The early 80's brought the aerobics craze. Racquetball clubs converted some of their courts into aerobics studios while other courts became equipment and free-weight rooms. With the introduction of the Lifecycle, computer technology made its way into the industry and brought fitness training to another level. New clubs were being built all across the country. In addition to the new clubs, existing clubs expanded and remodeled.

Bigger and better and why not— the economy boomed throughout the 80's and people were walking in the door and signing up left and right. Unfortunately, without much warning, the growth and prosperity of the early 80's came to a screeching halt by 1990.

* Source: International Health, Racquet & Sportsclub Association website.

Selling Fitness

The economy went into a recession. Many clubs, small and large, went out of business. Other clubs restructured, tightened their wallets and did whatever was necessary to make it through.

Consumers also made big changes. Gone were the days of frivolous spending. Consumers became much more selective, fully educating themselves about products and services before buying. They wanted the best value for their money. Consumers were in the drivers seat and businesses had to make the necessary adjustments.

One of the biggest adjustments was finding a new approach to selling. Strong closes and "today only" incentives were no longer tolerated. What is interesting is that consumers in the 90's demanded salespeople who were sincere, honest, and trustworthy. They looked for companies interested in long-term, service-driven relationships.

Now, two decades later, another economic slowdown and an even greater competitive market place for club operators means that good selling skills are more important than ever. Every prospect is important. Selling Fitness gives you step-by-step instructions on how to build quality relationships with every customer throughout the selling process.

The first half of Selling Fitness discusses how the technology of Neuro Linguistic Programming (NLP) applies to the selling of health and fitness memberships. NLP studies what drives human behavior and analyzes how our actions, both verbal and non-verbal, affect our interactions with others. The second half of Selling Fitness brings you, step-by-step, through the entire process of working with a guest. It covers everything from the initial phone contact to the post-sale referral and gives you cutting edge material that is specific to the needs and wants of fitness salespeople. Selling Fitness is designed for you to use as a desk reference throughout your selling career. I can only hope that this book provides you with the tools you need to be more productive and fulfilled while selling health and fitness memberships.

1

WHAT MOTIVATES PEOPLE TO BUY?

> *If you want to influence or affect what others do, you must have some understanding of the workings of human motivation-that force within us so powerful that it really decides what we do (or don't do)- how we do it- and why."*
>
> William Exton, Jr., <u>SELLING LEVERAGE</u>

When a customer walks through the front door and says, "I'm interested in getting a membership," why doesn't he always buy? Traditional training taught salespeople to ask some questions, find the customer's need and then fulfill that need with the company product or service. This approach sounds simple enough, but if that is all there is to sales, then why doesn't this logical method always work? All too often a sales person asks all the right questions, knows exactly what the customer wants, shows him how the club can fulfill those needs, and still no sale.

I remember the instance which made me realize that there had to be more to motivating someone to buy than what I had been taught. I was working membership sales when a guest walked into the club in an unusual way. Both glass doors had to be opened in order for him to fit! He was very open and candid about his obesity and poor fitness level. During the personal analysis, he admitted that his doctor had highly recommended a regular exercise program. Throughout the tour he gave positive responses to the usual tie-downs: "Do you think you can be here three days a week?," "What hours will you be using the club?" "Does the facility offer you enough variety?" etc. I thought, "This is an easy sale" moved on to the membership presentation and did not get a single objection. You can imagine how completely shocked I was when, after asking "Which is better for you, cash, check, or credit card?" this person tells me, "I need to think about it." Think about it! "Think about what?," I thought to myself. Nothing I said was going to change this person's mind and he left without joining. Here was someone who clearly had the need, was satisfied with what the facility had to offer, and did not have a problem with finances. I was frustrated. I wanted to know why he didn't walk out of the club as a happy new member.

In situations like this, as a defense mechanism, a convenience, or justification of a lost sale, salespeople often put the blame on the guest: "He wasn't serious," "He had an attitude," "He was just looking for some reason not to buy," or worse "He was just wasting my time." Granted, with the large numbers of people walking in and out of a facility one is sure to find a few guests who are not really serious. More accurately, most people who make the effort to come into a facility do have some interest in buying, <u>but leave because they were not motivated correctly</u>. What causes this to happen? More importantly, what can you do to prevent losing sales? Learning what motivates human behavior provides the foundation for a better understanding.

THE FORCES WITHIN YOU

Simply put, people do things for reasons. When one examines peoples' "reasons" for doing anything, <u>all human behavior can be traced back to two forces: The desire to gain pleasure and the need to avoid pain.</u> No matter how complex the reasons may appear, the underlying forces of pleasure and pain drive behavior.

What Motivates People To Buy?

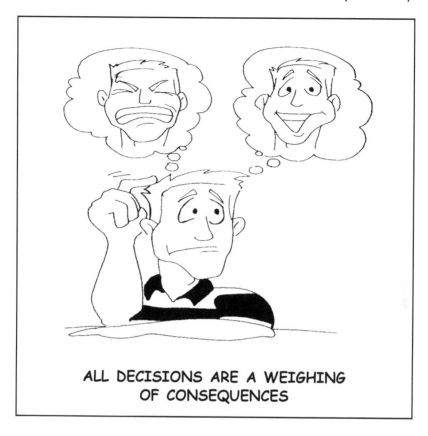

ALL DECISIONS ARE A WEIGHING OF CONSEQUENCES

Think about it; why do people diet? Some people diet to stay slim and look better, a form of pleasure they want to gain. Some people, however, don't diet for pleasure; they diet so they will not get fat, feel ashamed, embarrassed, and possibly ridiculed—all forms of pain they wish to avoid. Many times, though, behavior is the result of a combination of one wanting to gain pleasure and avoid pain.

Take, for example, getting up early to work out. Let's say that you set your alarm for 6 A.M. so you can exercise before going to work. Normally you get up at 7:30 A.M., but summer is coming and you want to get in shape. Basically your brain is saying, "Being in shape will make me feel better about myself," a form of pleasure. Before going to bed you get involved watching a movie and stay up late.

6 A.M. rolls around and the alarm rings. As you hit the snooze button you think, "Oh, just a few more minutes." The alarm rings again but your body doesn't want to get up. On one hand you are thinking, "I really should get up and go to the gym because I will feel better about myself" (pleasure) but on the other hand, "I'm tired from staying up late, and if I don't get more sleep I'll feel miserable all day at work." (pain). You decide to hit the snooze button again. The next time the alarm goes off you think, "I may feel miserable today, but just think how miserable I am going to feel when it's time to put on that bathing suit and I look like a marshmallow." (massive pain) All of a sudden, you bolt out of bed and speed off to the gym. The pain of being unattractive became greater than the pleasure of sleeping in late and that potential pain motivated you to take action.

Another example of the twin forces of pleasure and pain at work is when two friends tour a club together. One appears very interested, while the other isn't sure. What happens? Typically the dominant personality will have the greatest influence: If he says he is going to enroll, the less-assertive person will usually follow—even if he isn't completely sold on the idea—because the pain associated with not being "like" his friend is too great. On the other hand, if the dominant person says, "There is no way I'm going to buy today" the pain associated with buying and exercising alone is enough to influence the less-assertive person into an "I'd like to think about it" mode—even if he is ready to buy. Very rarely will one person buy that day if the other does not. This game of mental ping-pong between the forces of pleasure and pain is going on every moment of every day.

Think about a large purchase you made recently. How did you come to the decision to buy? Most likely, you didn't just wake up one day and say, "I want X," and immediately go out and buy it. What probably occurred was a thought process in which you considered all the pros and cons of that potential purchase. This period of consideration may have gone on for a few hours, days or months. Then, all of a sudden something clicked inside your brain and you made a decision.

What Motivates People To Buy?

No different than other decision-making processes, the buying process is a weighing of consequences. On one hand you have the pleasures of buying; on the other hand you have the pains. When one buys it is because he believes that the pleasure will outweigh the pain. If he doesn't, he believes that the pain will outweigh the pleasure. One important distinction is that **human beings will do much, much more to avoid pain than they will ever do to gain pleasure**. This distinction helps one to better understand why someone with medical problems may decide not to exercise. These people feel that the pain of exercising (and not just physical) is greater than the potential pain their medical problems may give them in the future and, as a result, will avoid the pain of exercising. For them it is a battle between two sources of pain, and they are looking for the lesser of two evils.

Now, you may say, "That's ridiculous, why would anyone want to jeopardize their own health?" Well why do people smoke when it is proven to cause cancer? Why doesn't someone who says "I really should quit this stinking habit" quit? Because, in his brain, the very real and *immediate* pain involved in the process of quitting is greater than the potential *distant* pain of possibly having cancer. Because the pain of cancer is not a reality (yet) it does not create motivation. Until something happens causing him to associate more pain to the potential consequences of smoking and less pain to the quitting process, he won't. Unfortunately, the same can be true with health and fitness. For someone to make life-style changes, it often takes something as serious as a heart attack, when they are faced with the very real pain of possibly dying.

Selling Fitness

USING THE FORCES IN SELLING

How does one go about using these two forces in the selling process? As we mentioned earlier, traditional sales taught salespeople to find the customer's need and then fulfill it with their product or service. This focused only on pleasure—the benefits of the purchase. Knowing that humans do much more to avoid pain than gain pleasure, good salespeople sell both types of consequences; the pleasure if they buy, and the pain if they don't.

Most salespeople, because of their positive nature, don't realize how important the element of pain is in the selling process. Elaborating on the painful consequences of not buying is sometimes the only way to get people motivated to do something for themselves.

For instance, if someone comes into your club one hundred pounds overweight and is about to walk out because he needs to "Think about it," <u>it is your job to respectfully get him to face the painful consequences of his obesity and motivate him to do something about it</u>. Don't nag or be rude—educate him about the benefits of exercising (pleasure) and the consequences of leading a sedentary life (pain). Next, give him a plan of action in the form of your product or service.

Advertisers have become masters at utilizing both forces of pleasure and pain. Take a television commercial where two good looking guys each drive onto the beach in their trucks. One guy has a cooler full of the "good" beer and the other guy has brand "X". Next, the guy with brand "X" is shown drinking alone while the guy with the "good brand" has a harem of beautiful women in bathing suits surrounding him. The commercial concludes when the guy drinking brand "X" leaves his beer behind, joins the others, ends up with the best looking woman at his side, and they all live happily ever after.

Advertisements do not come right out and say, "Buy our brand because it is better." A scene is created with a painful focus (no women) followed by a solution (the product). The result is an association that says, "Buy our beer and you will get beautiful women and have a good time." Even when the consumer logically knows that drinking a certain brand of beer is not going to give him women, the suggestions (both pro and con) are so powerful that the ad successfully motivates people to buy!

Another television commercial that clearly uses the two forces of pleasure and pain was put out by AT&T in the 1980's. The ad opens up with an elderly women sitting in her home with a sad look on her face. She stares at the phone and somberly says something like, "Wouldn't it be nice to hear from my son once in a while, but he is so busy he probably doesn't have time to call his mother"—clearly some major pain for any son. The next scene is a young man saying, "I think I'll call my mother." The screen flashes back to the mother picking up the phone and becoming ecstatic when she hears her son's voice, and then the jingle "Reach out, reach out and touch someone" resonates through the television. Everyone is happy and the son's guilt has been removed, at least until the next time he hears the ad!

Would the ad have been as effective if they just had the scene where the son calls his mother and she becomes all excited? Absolutely not! They first get the customer emotionally uncomfortable and feeling terribly guilty about the fact that he may not call his mother as often as he should. Once they have the customer feeling the pain, he is shown how he can heal that pain by simply picking up the phone and calling his mother. Consequently, the ad was one of the most successful. As one can see, when used correctly, the two forces of pain and pleasure can be used to compel a customer to take action.

DISSATISFACTION LEADS TO ACTION

 The bottom line is that in order to get a prospect to buy, you have to get him to a place of dissatisfaction: Feeling that he is not complete because he is not reaping the benefits of what your club has to offer. Focusing on just the potential satisfaction is not enough. He has to feel that his not buying is going to result in some form of emotional pain. Possibly he would be missing something or losing something. Maybe he would be alone, be inconvenienced or feel frustrated.

Although many salespeople, because of their positive nature, have a difficult time adjusting to selling the painful consequences instead of all the potential benefits, the initial level of discomfort is far less painful than watching potential sales walk out the door. Anyone who has sold memberships for even a short time can recall instances where they had "Mr. Congenial" as a guest. He is the type that during the tour says the facility is great and has everything he wants. Because he appears so content, showing no signs of reluctance, the salesperson skips over a lot of the usual question and answer stage assuming it will be an easy sale—until he gets to the close and Mr. Congenial says, "I need to think about it." Now the salesperson is stuck. The potential pleasure is not enough to motivate the guest to buy, but the salesperson has no idea what painful consequences this person wants to avoid.

As a last resort, many salespeople will start backtracking and asking the guest questions that focus on the painful consequences of them not buying: "You did say that you needed to get back in shape, how much longer are you going to wait? Isn't everyday that goes by only time lost?" The close is not the time to start this line of questioning; it is only perceived as a hard close and the guest may get angry and defensive. During the personal analysis and tour, quality time must be taken with every guest to determine the forces which are driving him.

What Motivates People To Buy?

Therefore, every guest who walks through the club doors without a signed check in hand should be treated as if he came to you for assistance. He has not determined why he wants to join and it is your job, your duty, to help him define his goals.

Of course, unless you want customers to walk out on you, one can't just come out and say, "I know you have this unconscious pain and it will go away if you buy this membership." Salespeople have to be as subtle as advertisers. No one wants to feel as if they are being sold. <u>Having the customer feel as if he is making the decision is a must.</u> Pushing someone into buying is manipulation. Getting someone to a place where he feels an **inner pressure** to buy is true motivation. When a guest has inner pressure he feels compelled to buy because it is what he wants to do—not because a salesperson has locked him up in a room and used one hundred and one "closes" until he finally gave-in and bought. Inner pressure is the most powerful tool for creating a shift in behavior and needs to be developed with respect and integrity. The customer's best interest must be kept in mind at all times.

Learning how to create that inner pressure within a prospect depends a great deal on knowing what a customer is buying when he purchases your products and services.

Selling Fitness

SUMMARY

1. All human behavior—motivation or lack thereof—can be traced back to two forces: The desire to gain pleasure and the need to avoid pain.

2. Human beings will do much more to avoid pain than they will to gain pleasure.

3. Good salespeople sell both types of consequences; the pleasure if the customer buys and the pain if they don't.

4. In order to get a prospect to buy, you have to get them to a place where they are experiencing a certain level of dissatisfaction with themself, either emotionally or physically.

5. Top salespeople get prospects to buy because they have created inner pressure within the customer, not because they are using external pressures.

EXERCISE

In effort to better understand how the elements of pleasure and pain play a role in your own motivation:

1. Remember a time you made a single purchase of $500 or more. What was it that motivated you to buy? Was it pleasure, pain, or a combination of the two? Write it down.

✎ _____
_____
_____
_____
_____

2. Remember a time that you wanted to make a large purchase but, when it came down to making the commitment, you decided against it. What were the pleasures that you wanted from having that product or service, and what were the painful consequences that prevented you from buying? Write them down.

✎ _____
_____
_____
_____
_____
_____

3. Remember, people will do much more to avoid pain than they will to gain pleasure. Therefore, it is important to have at least some elements of pain in your presentation. How can you professionally and respectfully incorporate some of the painful consequences of not exercising into your presentation? Are there any statistics that would be helpful? Any materials or fact sheets that could be used during your presentation?

2

WHAT DO PEOPLE BUY?

> *We should think of ourselves as being in the connection business, or the feeling-good business. People don't really need to belong to a club in order to work out, get healthy and fit. They can do that on their own at much less cost.* ***They belong because they like to be around other people, especially people who make them feel good****...People are more responsive to feelings than to reason... They are drawn to what they enjoy. It's time for us to start thinking of our clubs as places of fun, of joy.*
>
> Warren Wertheimer, owner, Rolling Hills Club

What type of automobile do you drive? Is it American or an import? Sporty, rugged, luxurious? Is it red, silver, white, blue? Although I have never tried counting, there must be 75-100 different brands and styles of cars available. When one combines that with color and other options there must be hundreds of choices available. Even within certain price ranges there are dozens of choices, *so what made you choose the one you did?* I mean a car is a car; they all have four wheels, an engine, and get you from point A to point B, right? If that is the case, then why wouldn't I be caught dead driving an Aries K car—even when I had the chance to inherit one free of charge? Because the reality of the situation is that although we buy a product because we have a need for it (I needed a car to get to work), driving certain makes, models, and colors produces within each one of us different feelings. How would you feel driving down the street in a 540 SL

Selling Fitness

Mercedes? Whatever your feelings would be, I bet they would be different than if you were driving an Aries K car. I drive a Rodeo (and now have a car payment) because, unlike the Aries K car, the Rodeo gives me the feelings of being a sporty-outdoors type; both are feelings I want.

PEOPLE BUY WANTS

The fact is that people do not buy needs. People buy wants, and wants are emotional, not logical or rational. The auto industry does not get people to spend $80,000 on a car because it is logical or rational. No one needs an $80,000 car. They want a certain car because having it will give them a particular feeling; a feeling they think is worth spending $80,000 to get. Through the years, the advertising industry has become masters at conditioning people to link products with emotions: Drive a Mercedes and you get prestige; drive a Pontiac and you get excitement; drive a Ford truck and you are American-tough; drive a Volvo wagon and you get intelligent security.

What is amazing is that advertisers have gotten us to link completely different feelings to products that are essentially the same. Car manufacturers take the same basic components, put a different style body over the top of it, put a new name on the fender, create a high powered advertising campaign and, like magic, they have a new product to sell. We, as consumers, want the feelings that have been linked to the product. Therefore, when a customer walks through your club doors and is considering purchasing a membership, you must remember <u>he is not buying the pool, the weights, and the aerobic classes which he needs to exercise. He is buying the emotions he will experience as a result of using those products and services</u>. You must sell the emotional wants, not just the facilities needed to work out in.

24

What Do People Buy?

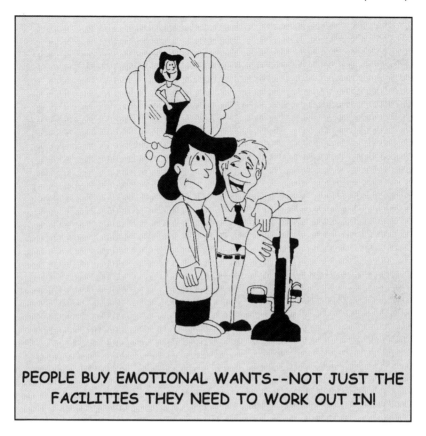

PEOPLE BUY EMOTIONAL WANTS--NOT JUST THE FACILITIES THEY NEED TO WORK OUT IN!

THE CHALLENGE

Of course, your job would be a breeze if selling emotional wants was as easy as discussing it. The challenge to you is that emotional wants happen at the unconscious level. Guests do not walk into the club and say, "I really want to feel more self confident and I think I can accomplish that by getting into shape." Instead, guests come in focused on the facility and will tell you, "I want a nice pool which has extended hours." In order to make your presentation appeal to the guest at a deep level— getting him motivated to buy—you will have to "uncover" what his emotional wants are. Therefore, when he tells you he wants a nice pool with extended hours, you need to find out what that means to him. The "uncovering process might go something like this:

Selling Fitness

Guest: I want a nice pool with extended hours.

You: The extended hours are important to you because...?

Guest: Because I want to be able to come in even when my schedule is hectic.

You: Was that a problem for you at your last club?

Guest: Yes.

You: What happened? Or, What was the result?

Guest: I couldn't be consistent with my workouts and stay in shape all year long.

You: So, staying in shape all year long is important to you?

Guest: Very important because at my age it is not that easy to drop 4 or 5 pounds.

You: I'm curious, does consistently staying in shape have an affect on how you feel about yourself?

Guest: Oh, definitely; I think I have more energy and feel more confident.

Although it may take more conversation than this example to get all this information, the result will be digging deeper to find out what he wants at an emotional level. Even if the guest does not give you something as specific as "self-confidence," you will have gained valuable information. Remember the forces of pleasure and pain? In this example, the guest indicated what was motivating him before he got specific. First, he said that, "Losing 4 or 5 pounds was not as easy as it used to be," a potential pain he wants to avoid. Second, he said that staying in shape all year long gave him more energy and made him feel more self confident, definitely a form of pleasure he wants to have.

What Do People Buy?

By asking questions which help to uncover a guest's real wants and then carefully listening to what he says, you will obtain valuable information which can be used throughout your tour and presentation.

WANTS ARE AN INDIVIDUAL THING

Take ten people who all say that having money is important to them and ask, "So, what does having money give you emotionally?" Chances are you will get ten different responses. To one person having money gives them prestige, to another it's security, and to another it's independence. What is important to one person may not have even entered another's mind. That is because wants are a very individual thing. Therefore, when someone tells you that he wants a nice pool with extended hours, you have no idea what that ultimately means to him. You need to ask the right questions to uncover his emotional wants. This will be covered in more detail in chapter 7, The Personal Analysis.

CONFLICTING WANTS

One final factor that you must keep in mind is that people can have conflicting wants which results in self-sabotage. Suppose that an overweight individual comes into the club. He has a long history of ups and downs with his weight. He says what he wants most from his membership is to lose weight and keep it off—moving towards self-worth. Failure is the feeling he wants to avoid. Human behavior indicates that he will do much more to avoid the failure than to gain the self-worth. Therefore, your job will be to direct the conversation so that he associates that not trying would make him feel like more of a failure than if he tried and did not succeed. Unless you successfully do this, he will not buy.

Selling Fitness

SUMMARY

1. People do not buy needs, they buy wants.

2. The challenge in sales is uncovering the prospect's emotional wants.

3. Wants are an individual thing: One person may say they want a nice pool with extended hours which ultimately gives them the feeling of more self confidence. Another person may want the same pool with extended hours, which ultimately allows them to avoid the humiliation of being out of shape.

4. Sometimes people have conflicting wants which can result in self-sabotage.

EXERCISE

Take a moment to uncover your own emotional wants for exercising. Ask yourself, "What does exercising give me/do for me" and continue to do so until you finally get to a feeling or emotion.

Example:

I exercise because I like to have a firm body.

Which allows me to look good in whatever I wear.

Which makes me feel more attractive and confident. (pleasure)
Or
Which means I won't be ashamed of my body. (pain)

✎ Write your answer down:

_____
_____
_____
_____
_____
_____
_____
_____

3

WHY BUY FROM YOU?

> *Faced with no discernible difference in products, what buyers are looking for are salespeople who have their clients' interest at heart.*
>
> Larry Wilson, CHANGING THE GAME

Right now, get your phone book. Open it up to the yellow pages under "Health Clubs." How many clubs other than yours are listed? Unless you live in a secluded area, there is probably more than one club offering a comparable product at a competitive price. Compound that with the fact that the economy is not what it was in the 80's and what you get are consumers who are much more selective and reluctant to spend money. So, what is going to make a customer buy from you instead of a competitor? You make the difference! You need to do things that are going to make you shine brighter than the rest of your competition.

AN ATTITUDE ADJUSTMENT

The first thing that will separate you from other salespeople is your attitude. The attitude you project, both verbally and non-verbally, is a direct result of your beliefs and perceptions about your job. If you think that your job is just selling memberships, your attitude will reflect that. You need to stop thinking of yourself strictly as a salesperson and start thinking of yourself as a "Lifestyle Consultant;" someone who helps others! As minor as that change may sound, it will have a huge impact on the attitude you project.

Selling Fitness

Another element of attitude is how you perceive your prospects. Because most fitness salespeople earn the bulk of their income from commissions, over time you may stop thinking of prospects as human beings with needs and wants and start seeing them in terms of how many dollars their purchase will net for you. This is a sure fire way to start losing sales. Ask any salesperson who has entered into a prospective sale in the "desperate for a commission mode" how successful they were, and 99% of them will tell you that they did not make the sale. One way to avoid this pitfall is to ask yourself three questions before talking to or greeting any new prospect:

1. I wonder what I will like about this guest?

2. I wonder if this guest will become a good friend?

3. How can I help this guest get what he wants?

By asking yourself these simple questions, you will put yourself into a frame of mind that will project a positive, sincere attitude. The guest will sense this and will be more likely to open up to you as a friend. And remember, people are more comfortable and willing to buy from friends! If you think of your guests as friends and come from a place where, in your heart, you really want to make a difference in the quality of their lives, I guarantee that you will make more sales and have more fun and fulfillment doing it.

EXCEED EXPECTATIONS

Another way that you can distinguish yourself from other salespeople is by constantly exceeding the prospect's expectations. As you may already know, the general public has made gross generalizations about salespeople. They figure that salespeople are going to be nice to them until they don't buy, and then they expect the salesperson to get pushy and unpleasant with them.

Make sure that you do not give prospects any reason to believe that this common misconception is true. No matter what a prospect says or does—even if he is rude to you—always be pleasant and polite with him. Do the unexpected; always send a thank you note, even if he does not buy. <u>By constantly exceeding expectations, your prospect will realize that you want to build long term relationships and are willing to work with him until he is ready to buy.</u>

STAYING POWER

In addition to exceeding expectations prior to the sale, you must not forget that the question, "Why should I buy from you" is an ongoing one. The days of "lifetime" memberships are over. Most memberships are one year programs with options to cancel after that time. In order to get a member to want to keep buying from you—year after year—you must maintain quality relationships. A member must feel that you have their best interest in mind at all times! Therefore, frequent personal contact is a must. Regular phone calls just to say "Hi, how is everything? Can I do anything for you? Do you need anything?" are another way to separate yourself from other salespeople and create long-term members.

ANCHORING

Is there someone in your life who, the minute you see or hear from them you get totally happy? You could be having a miserable day but the instant you hear their voice or see their face, you smile and, for a while, forget that you were having such a bad day? Maybe you know someone who does just the opposite to you. That is, you could be having a great day and at the mention of their name or the sight of their face you snarl, feel lousy or maybe even get angry? When you associate feelings and emotions with another person to the degree that you instantly experience those feelings and emotions the minute you think about, hear, or see that individual, your brain has created, what

Selling Fitness

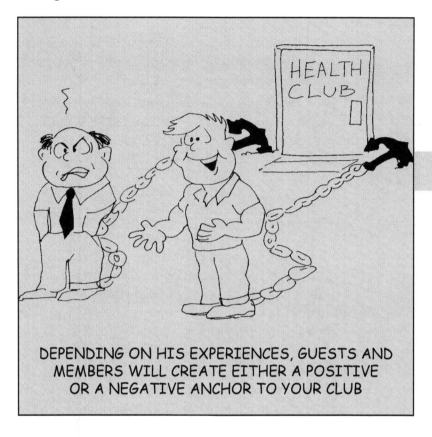

DEPENDING ON HIS EXPERIENCES, GUESTS AND MEMBERS WILL CREATE EITHER A POSITIVE OR A NEGATIVE ANCHOR TO YOUR CLUB

Neuro Linguistic Programming refers to as, an *anchor*. Meaning that your brain has linked those feeling and emotions to that person. X person = happiness; Y person = hostility.

Every minute of everyday your brain is creating and re-creating anchors. For example, say that you are in the market for a new car. Because an advertiser did a good job of getting you to anchor certain feelings and emotions to a particular make and model, you go out and purchase that car. You are on top of the world driving around in your new vehicle. Because you are positively anchored to it, every time you see the car you feel great. Let's say, though, that after a few weeks your car breaks down and has to be towed to the dealership. You are not pleased but you are more concerned about getting the car fixed. You breathe a sigh of relief when the serviceman says, "All set, it's as good as new."

Just when you are happy to be back in you new car it breaks down again. You go from concerned to annoyed. By the third time it breaks down, you are down right angry! Now, when you look at what is supposed to be your nice new car, all you want to do is put it in gear and let it drop off a cliff. What happened? As you continued to have problems, your brain created a new association. The result is having a negative anchor attached to your car.

This process of creating and recreating anchors with a car can also happen with people. You begin to date someone and fall madly in love. Anytime you hear his voice or see his face you get goose bumps. As time goes by you have a few disagreements but you figure that is to be expected. What were just disagreements, though, soon turn into full fledged arguments. After a while, the two of you can not even talk on the phone without having the conversation escalate into a yelling match. A good friend who has not spoken to you since you first fell in love calls and says, "How is _____ ?" Your body gets tense, you get a disgusted look on your face and you sarcastically say, "That loser!" What was once a positive anchor that produced goose bumps is now a negative anchor that produces a feeling of disgust.

How does all this apply to selling? Simply put, whether you like it or not, prospects are creating and recreating anchors to you and the club every time they walk through the doors or talk to you on the phone. <u>If you do not get prospects anchored positively to you and the club from the very beginning of your relationship, you are going to have a very difficult time getting them to buy from you</u>. One of the keys to creating positive anchors with others is having a good level of rapport with them. Let us move on to the next chapter and find out exactly what rapport is.

SUMMARY

1. With many competitors selling the same product at a comparable price, you make the difference.

2. You must have the attitude that your job is not just selling memberships, but that you are a "Lifestyle Consultant" who is helping others get what they want.

3. Make sure that you always see prospects as human beings with needs and wants, not just in terms of dollars to you. One way to ensure this is by asking yourself three questions before talking or greeting any new prospect:

- ✓ I wonder what I will like about this guest?
- ✓ I wonder if this guest will become a good friend?
- ✓ How can I help this guest get what he wants?

4. In order to set yourself apart from other salespeople, continually exceed expectations: Always being polite and sending thank you notes are two ways to do that.

5. Having the right attitude and exceeding expectations has to be the way you do business 365 days a year, not just something you do until the sale is made.

6. Remember, a prospect is creating and recreating anchors to you every time he walks through the doors or speaks to you on the phone. Make sure you are giving him reasons to have a positive anchor!

EXERCISE

Think of a time that you purchased something which involved a relationship with a salesperson where:

A) You had a choice of two or more places to buy the same or similar products from and; B) All of the places had comparable prices.

What made you buy where you did? Did one salesperson do something over and above all the others or did one or more of the salespeople do something which angered you enough to buy from the other? Take the time to think about it then write your answer below.

4

RAPPORT & COMMUNICATION STYLES

> *I know there's a myth flying around somewhere that opposites attract. But let me tell you this: When the initial challenge of opposite attraction wears off, we're left with someone who thinks, acts, and behaves unlike what we consider the norm.*
>
> Michael Brooks, INSTANT RAPPORT

Two guests simultaneously walk into the club. Person A has a bounce in his step; he approaches the front desk with a smile and enthusiastically says, "Hi, I would like to find out about your memberships." Person B moves at a much slower pace. He is looking down and when he finally reaches the front desk you can barely make out his soft-spoken words; "I wanted to find out about your memberships." You are scheduled to work with the next walk-in. Who are you going to choose to work with? I have yet to find a salesperson who, knowing nothing about rapport technology, says they would pick person B. Why is it that just because someone is not doing cartwheels as they walk through the front door a salesperson would choose not to work with them?

WHAT IS RAPPORT?

What is it that attracts you to some people and not to others? The answer is rapport. Of course, the idea of establishing rapport is nothing new to sales. If someone does not like or trust another, the chances of the customer buying from that person are greatly reduced. Traditional sales training (and "social skills" in general) teach that in order to establish rapport one must "get to know" his customer. How one does that is to ask a lot of questions; the strategy is to get the customer talking so they open up. Obviously, this approach is not all that bad because most salespeople use it and millions of products are sold every day. Haven't you had those instances, though, when you asked all the questions and the customer did not open up? When you finished with the personal analysis you felt as though you still knew little or nothing about them. What causes this to happen? Those willing to examine rapport from a different perspective found that the questions themselves do not establish the rapport. Rather, the level of commonality that one felt—verbally and non-verbally—as a result of the questions, was responsible for creating that bond. Simply stated, **rapport is nothing but a feeling of commonality**. People are attracted to people who are like them. Do you spot a punk-rocker with a spiked, purple hair cut, leather jacket, chains and a tattoo and wonder what it would take to get a date with that person? Another punk-rocker would. When people feel as if they have something in common, they begin to feel a bond. This bond is what creates a feeling of rapport and an unconscious desire to respond.

Rapport is the foundation for good communication. It is so easy to talk to someone you like. The real challenge begins when one is forced to communicate with someone they do not feel comfortable with, especially when they do not know why. When choosing friends, one may be in control of whom they wish to affiliate, but professionally few people have that option. As a salesperson, no doubt, you have had to work with someone whom you did not wish to interact, someone you would have liked to avoid at all costs—someone who is not "like you." At such times, understanding communication styles becomes imperative.

COMMUNICATION STYLES

If rapport is nothing but a feeling of commonality, understanding what makes people feel uncommon or different from one another is a must. Aside from external factors such as appearance and physical attributes, one of the fundamental differences between human beings is their communication style. There are three primary types of communicators: Visual, auditory, and kinesthetic.

All information from the external world is taken in through the senses. Although everyone utilizes all of their senses, each person has a preference for one sense over the others. Knowing those preferences is the key to establishing rapport. Once someone's sensory preference is known, certain reactions and behaviors can be anticipated. By identifying the visual, auditory, or kinesthetic personality you will be able to create that feeling of commonality, hence rapport, by communicating in the manner that is most comfortable and understandable to your client.

SPOTTING THE VISUAL COMMUNICATOR

This guest walks through the club doors quickly. Upon entering his eyes are busy looking at everything he can possibly see. He quickly finds the front desk and says to the receptionist, "I would like to take a *look* at the facility." Even after being instructed to have a seat on the couch while a salesperson is located, this guest can't be bothered with sitting. Instead, he continues to walk around taking in all the sights—he may even attempt to enter the work-out area because he is so eager to *see* the facility. Prepare yourself for the visual guest.

A visual communicator receives and sorts out information (learning) primarily by creating pictures in his mind. Similarly, when a visual person is pulling information from his brain's files,

Selling Fitness

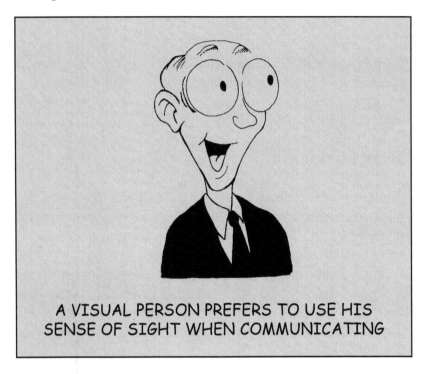

A VISUAL PERSON PREFERS TO USE HIS SENSE OF SIGHT WHEN COMMUNICATING

(remembering) he does so in the form of pictures and consequently, tries to give out or communicate information by creating pictures to the person with whom he is speaking. Therefore, directions given by visual person will sound like this: "Take a left at the second light. Go through one stop sign. You will go past a small white house with blue shutters and directly across from the yellow school-crossing sign is the community center." Ask a visual person for street names and he probably won't know, even if it is a street he travels frequently. "Don't worry," he will say; "You can't miss it; it's the street with the convenience store on one corner and the hair salon on the other." The visual person has made pictures of the surroundings and its landmarks, and the street names are not of primary importance. A visual person knows he is in the right place when "it looks right" to him. Another example of a visual's behavior is the way he shops. Visual people don't make lists when they go to the grocery store. They just walk through the aisles knowing they will *see* what items are needed. As a result, visuals have a tendency to forget things, such as the cheese for tonight's pizza because they didn't walk past the dairy case!

Rapport & Communication Styles

A visual person's speech patterns are extremely fast because pictures are worth what? That's right, a thousand words! Pictures are flashing in and out of the visual person's brain so quickly that his words cannot keep up with the pictures. As a result, visual people are not concerned with how they sound when speaking. They don't have enough time to carefully choose the words that would best describe the pictures that are flashing through their brain. By the time they have found the best word, the picture has gone and they have drawn a "total blank." In fact, a visual person's explanations to a non-visual person can be rather amusing—even frustrating. He will keep trying to explain the pictures he sees in his mind and will say things like: "Well, you *see*, it's like this...." When he *sees*, by the expression on your face, that you did not understand, he will start again, "*Picture* it this way...," and off he'll go. Quite often a visual person won't understand his own explanation. He may go through an intense description only to say, "No, no, that isn't right; imagine it like this...." Then he will look at you and say, "Can't you *see* that?" "Is that *clear*?" In addition to the fast pace at which visuals speak, the words they use indicate that they are visualizing. Below is a list of words and phrases frequently utilized by someone in a visual mode. Hearing the words and phrases provides you with the clues you need to "spot the visual."

SEE	LOOK	VIEW
APPEAR	SHOW	DAWN
REVEAL	ENVISION	ILLUMINATE
TWINKLE	CLEAR	FOGGY
FOCUSED	HAZY	SPARKLING
FLASH	IMAGINE	

AN EYEFUL	BEYOND A SHADOW
BIRD'S EYE VIEW	CATCH A GLIMPSE OF
CLEAR CUT	CRYSTAL CLEAR
DIM VIEW	EYE TO EYE
FLASHED ON	GET A SCOPE ON

Selling Fitness

HAZY IDEA	IN LIGHT OF
IN PERSON	IN VIEW OF
LOOKS LIKE	MAKE A SCENE
MENTAL IMAGE	MENTAL PICTURE
MIND'S EYE	NAKED EYE
PAINT A PICTURE	PLAINLY SEE
PRETTY AS A PICTURE	SEE TO IT
SHOWING OFF	STARING OFF INTO
SPACE	SHORTSIGHTED
TAKE A PEEK	TUNNEL VISION
GET A PERSPECTIVE OF	
PHOTOGRAPHIC MEMORY	

The personal analysis offers the perfect opportunity to determine someone's communication style. Since visual people are concerned with how they look, when asked why they wish to start an exercise program, most will say they want to look better or continue to look good. Finally, the visual guest will give you an indication of whether or not he is going to enroll by saying "Well, it looks like the club has everything I will need", or "I did not see a sauna or a whirlpool, do you have one?"

Body movement will also indicate the mode in which someone is communicating. Visual people don't just speak quickly, they move quickly. The pace at which they walk is fast, and they are often described as, "Always being in a hurry." In addition, visual people use hand gestures while speaking—not just small, contained movements, but large, circular, sweeping, movements. Being with a visual person who is getting ready to go out is like watching a movie in fast forward! As he rushes out the door, he realizes he has forgotten something and turns around so rapidly that you find yourself smashing into him. He may run in and out of the house two or three times before he has everything.

Rapport & Communication Styles

Although a more subtle element, a person's breathing is also an excellent indicator of a person's mode. Breathing has a tremendous impact on rapport because it is biofeedback at the deepest level—existence! When someone is in a visual mode, breathing is high in his chest. He takes shallow breaths because he doesn't have time to breathe deeply.

Although a gross generalization, a majority of the people working in the health and fitness industry are visual people. Fast, energetic, enthusiastic individuals who have the ability to endure the worst possible morning—oversleep; no time for a shower; fix a flat tire on the way to work—and still smile saying, "Good morning, isn't it a great day?" the minute members walk through the door.

HEARING THE AUDITORY COMMUNICATOR

Unlike the visual, an auditory person enters the club and immediately finds the front desk. Why? To *talk* to someone, of course! "I would like to *talk* to someone about memberships," he says. Rarely in a hurry and not concerned with how something looks, the auditory person will follow the receptionist's instructions and sit down in the waiting area. He will usually pick-up any brochures, magazines, or information that may be near him because reading text is the process of hearing himself talk.

For and auditory person, listening is everything. When information is taken into his brain, instead of making pictures as visual people do, an auditory person will retain the information via words and sounds. How would he give directions? "This is Main Street. Follow Main Street approximately 1.5 miles; when you cross over Lake Street the first street on your left is Lexington Avenue. There is a traffic light there. You will go through one stop sign, approximately 1/4 of a mile, and the community center is on your left." The auditory person knows street names and numbers because these are his points of reference. If you ask him for landmarks (a visual ques-

Selling Fitness

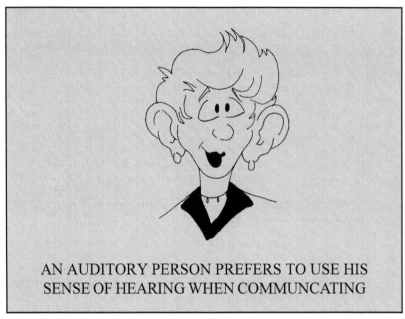

AN AUDITORY PERSON PREFERS TO USE HIS SENSE OF HEARING WHEN COMMUNCATING

tion), he will *tell* you not to worry, "The street sign clearly says Lexington Ave." The auditory person is a thinker. He wants to get things right the first time. He frequently has some sort of appointment book or "things to do" note pad and actually uses them. When shopping, the auditory person will always make a list and check it twice. Unlike the visual person, he won't have to go back to the store for the pizza cheese, he will have it every time!

Because how things *sound* is of primary importance. The auditory person speaks much slower than the visual person. He takes the time to think about what he is going to say before saying it. This is in sharp contrast to the visual person who blurts out words until they finally make sense. The words and phrases used by an auditory person clearly indicate that he processes the world around him with sounds. Below is a list of words and phrases commonly used by the auditory person.

HEAR	LISTEN	SOUND(S)
HARMONIZE	DEAF	SILENCE
RESONATE	MELLIFLUOUS	DISSONANCE
ATTUNE	OVERTONES	QUESTION

Rapport & Communication Styles

EARFUL	OUTSPOKEN
UTTERLY	TUNE IN/OUT
BE ALL EARS	RINGS A BELL
BE HEARD	UNHEARD-OF
AFTER-THOUGHT	BLABBER-MOUTH
CLEAR AS A BELL	CLEARLY EXPRESSED
CALL ON	DESCRIBE IN DETAIL
MAKE MUSIC	EXPRESS YOURSELF
GIVE AN ACCOUNT OF	GIVE ME YOUR EAR
GRANT AN AUDIENCE	HEARD VOICES
HOLD YOUR TONGUE	IDLE TALK
INQUIRE INTO	KEY-NOTE SPEAKER
LOUD AND CLEAR	MANNER OF SPEAKING
PAY ATTENTION TO	POWER OF SPEECH
PURRS LIKE A KITTEN	RAP SESSION
TATTLE TALE	TO TELL THE TRUTH
TONGUE TIED	VOICE AN OPINION
STATE YOUR PURPOSE	

<u>During the personal analysis, the auditory communicator may say something like, "I have been *thinking* about this for some time and I finally *said* to myself, you have to stop procrastinating."</u> The auditory person is not so concerned with how the club looks, as finding answers to all his questions about facilities, services, and programs. In his mind, he must get all these questions answered. One can tell whether the auditory person approves of the club because he will say, "This *sounds* like a good program", or, "I *think* this will work out."

Like their speech patterns, the body movements of auditory people are also slower than those of the visuals. Auditory people think things out before they take action. This results in less running around to get things accomplished. In getting ready to go out, an auditory person will make a mental checklist before he goes out the door. "Let me *think*; I've done this, that, this and that. Okay, all ready to go." It is unusual for an auditory person to run in and out of the door five times before leaving. In addition, his hand gestures are smaller and more contained than those of the visuals. He often stands with his arms crossed in front of him or one hand on his chin in a "thinking position."

Because someone in an auditory mode is not in such a rush as the visual person, his breathing is from the middle of the abdomen. In addition, he has a much more regular and rhythmic pattern of breathing. When *thinking* about his response, an auditory person will often take a deep breath in and exhale a *sigh* before responding.

GRASPING THE KINESTHETIC

The kinesthetic guest quietly approaches the front desk and patiently awaits the receptionist to greet him. He will say, "I would like to *find out* more about your facility" in what appears to visual and auditory communicators as showing half-hearted interest. He is not bouncing through the doors with outwardly expressed excitement. While content taking a seat in the waiting area, he has a chance to get a *feel* for the atmosphere of the club. As with most unfamiliar territory, expect that it may take the kinesthetic a while to feel comfortable.

Instead of making pictures or hearing sounds, the kinesthetic person processes his world and retains information through feelings, emotions, tactile sensations (sense of touch), or proprioreceptors (sense of movement). When a kinesthetic person gives directions, however, he is forced to use pictures and words. This results in the directions being given slowly. He will stop to think for a long time, wondering if his directions are "the best way." He has to *feel* as though he has given the directions correctly, and it takes much longer to process feelings than it does pictures or words. The kinesthetic shopper is in no hurry. He will make a list and still go down each aisle carefully, getting a *sense* for anything he may have forgotten to write down. He may also leave with more in the shopping cart than he planned because coming across a particular product may have given him a craving that had to be fulfilled.

Rapport & Communication Styles

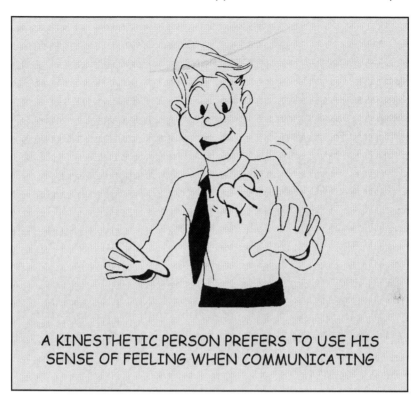

A KINESTHETIC PERSON PREFERS TO USE HIS SENSE OF FEELING WHEN COMMUNICATING

Because he goes inside himself to get a feeling for what he is going to say before he says it, the kinesthetic person speaks much more slowly than a visual or auditory person. Sometimes, when speaking with a kinesthetic person or asking him a question, you may begin to think that he is either not listening or not going to answer because he might take a minute or more before responding. Many auditory and particularly visual people have a tendency to lose patience when speaking with kinesthetic people. This is unfortunate because kinesthetic people have a lot to offer; they are very caring and compassionate people and can provide opinions and points of view that are extremely important. Generally, kinesthetic people tend to speak softly. Once again, this causes some discomfort to the visual and auditory communicators because they have difficulty hearing the kinesthetic person and impatiently ask him to repeat himself. Below is a list of words and phrases commonly used by kinesthetic people.

Selling Fitness

FEEL	TOUCH
GRASP	HARD
UNFEELING	CONCRETE
SCRAPE	SOLID
SUFFER	GET HOLD OF
SLIP THROUGH	TAP INTO
MAKE CONTACT	THROW OUT
TURN AROUND	STUBBORN
GET A HANDLE ON IT	SLIPPED MY MIND
ALL WASHED UP	BOILS DOWN TO
CONTROL YOURSELF	HOLD IT!
CHIP OFF THE OLD BLOCK	COME TO GRIPS WITH
FIRM FOUNDATIONS	HAND IN HAND
FLOATING ON THIN AIR	GET A LOAD OF THIS
GET IN TOUCH WITH	GET THE DRIFT OF
HANG IN THERE	HEATED ARGUMENT
HOLD ON!	

HOT HEAD	KEEP YOUR SHIRT ON
KNOW-HOW	LAY CARDS ON TABLE
MOMENT OF PANIC	NOT FOLLOWING YOU
PAIN-IN-THE-NECK	PULL SOME STRINGS
SHARP AS A TACK	START FROM SCRATCH
\SO-SO	STIFF UPPER LIP
COOL/CALM/COLLECTED	

<u>During the personal analysis, the kinesthetic guest will reply that the reason he came in was to *feel* better or to *get a hold of* his weight problem.</u> They will use words like *feel*, and *sense*, and have at tendency to use metaphors. It is important to remember that the kinesthetic person will want to take his time making a decision because he wants to make sure that it feels right. This may require a full work-out or even an additional visit before he is willing to make a commitment.

Because he processes the world around him through feelings, and accessing feelings does not require a lot of movement, kinesthetic people are not as physically expressive as the visual and auditory communicators. In fact, kinesthetic people enjoy many things that do not require a lot of physical activity. This is not to say that they don't enjoy physical activity—they do—they are just more laid back than the visual and auditory communicators and, as a result, are also content doing slower paced activities. Consequently, when speaking, the kinesthetic person does not make many hand gestures or body movements. Very frequently, he will fidget with something during the conversation, appearing to be more focused on that object than on you. The object could be anything from a pen or paper clip, to the cuff of his sleeve, to his own hands, and is not meant as an insult to auditory and visual communicators; it serves only as something for the kinesthetic person to *grab on to* while he sorts through his feelings. The kinesthetic person does not run around or need a list when getting ready to go out, he intuitively knows that he has everything.

The kinesthetic person breathes from his lower abdomen at a slow, consistent pace. Before responding to a question requiring any type of thought or opinion, the kinesthetic person will take a very deep breath and exhale slowly, followed by a long, silent pause allowing him to get in touch with what he is feeling in regards to the question.

The kinesthetic person is the most underrated prospect for sales, particularly in the health and fitness industry. Kinesthetic people's calmness is often interpreted as indifference. The kinesthetic guest, however, is sometimes the easiest type of person to motivate because he is already in touch with the feelings and emotions that are really driving a person to buy. When one says to a kinesthetic person "Well, how would you feel about yourself if you didn't get started on an exercise program," he easily gets associated with that question. Visual and auditory guests may think this line of questioning is just a sales tactic. To the kinesthetic it probably will not be taken that way.

AUDITORY DIGITAL

There is one more category of communicator which represents a very small percentage of the population; auditory-digital. Auditory-digital people process information with facts and figures-digital information. In addition to the basic characteristics of auditory people, auditory-digital people actually want those charts and brochures displayed at the car dealership explaining the features! They want the bottom line and often speak in percentages. An auditory digital person may respond, "I'm not one hundred percent today, I'm only about eighty-seven percent." Eighty-seven percent of what, one wonders? Percentages, facts, and figures—these are what the auditory-digital person demands. Imagine how difficult an auditory-digital style of communication can be for a visuals mind to comprehend—how do you make a picture of eighty-seven percent!

In the health and fitness industry, auditory-digital people have a tendency to drive salespeople crazy. The auditory-digital person appears to be interested but asks so many seemingly irrelevant questions that the salesperson becomes impatient. "What percentage of your members use the facility after 5pm?" "What is the ratio of active to inactive members?"; and the all time favorite, "Would it be okay if I took a copy of the agreement home with me before I signed it?" It is very difficult for others to understand how someone could be so hung up about details. Remember, although most people wouldn't even think to ask these questions, details of this nature are of primary concern to the auditory-digital communicator.

KEEPING THINGS IN PERSPECTIVE

 It must be kept in mind that the preceding scenarios are generalizations. Saying someone is visual, auditory, or kinesthetic is a convenience which allows you to better understand the communication process. Consequently, you may know someone who does not really fit into any of these categories; no one is exclusively any one particular type of communicator. Every person utilizes all three types of com-

Rapport & Communication Styles

munication styles in his day-to-day living, but each of us tends to prefer one of the three types as our primary mode.

Knowing the attributes of the three basic types of communicators enables you to recognize your own preferences and with practice, what others' preferences are. Let's find out how these styles affect your interactions with others and the level of rapport—or lack of—that is attained. Comparing the different interactions will show much more clearly how such differences can make or break communication.

Interaction between a visual person and a kinesthetic person can be extremely frustrating for both. Remember, visual people talk and move very quickly, while kinesthetic people talk and move quite slowly. What happens? From the visual person's point of view, the kinesthetic person in unmotivated, insecure, and boring. Even worse, the visual person has to keep asking for answers to be repeated because of the kinesthetic person's soft voice. Indeed, the visual person will probably try to complete the kinesthetic's sentences for him because he speaks so slowly. The kinesthetic person quite rightly resents being treated as if he's not smart enough to finish his own sentences, not realizing that he is literally going inside himself and sorting out how he feels about the situation before responding. Everybody takes longer to sort out feelings, it just happens to be how the kinesthetic person communicates most of the time. A visual person may mention that he finds someone nice but boring because he, "never seems to want to have any fun, he just wants to hang out." Unfortunately for the visual person, he has just destroyed any rapport with the kinesthetic person because "hanging out" with someone is what kinesthetic types enjoy most.

From a kinesthetic perspective, visual people come across as loud and obnoxious. For him, haste makes waste, and visual people are too hasty. Visual people talk so fast that the kinesthetic's brain literally cannot process all the information he is receiving fast enough since processing feelings takes a lot longer than creating pictures. How

Selling Fitness

does a kinesthetic person feel about a visual person? He probably finds him to be nice enough but in too much of a hurry. The kinesthetic person often feels he can never get a word in edgewise. He may be hurt by the visual's lack of patience.

As mentioned earlier, the majority of people in the health and fitness industry fall into visual and "high" auditory categories. When hiring, clubs want outwardly enthusiastic people who enjoy talking, interacting and motivating. Unfortunately, because of the perception that kinesthetic people are unmotivated, salespeople have a tendency to drive kinesthetic people out the door. The salesperson talks and moves so fast that he feels as though he will never remember all that he has to do. Kinesthetic people often admit that the club is, "too much for them to handle."

What about an auditory person interacting with a visual person? How much confidence would an auditory person have with directions given by a visual person? The auditory would probably perceive the visual person as incompetent and find it hard to believe that the guy lives in the town, works at the gas station, and doesn't know the names of streets! On the other hand, the visual person getting directions from an auditory person will constantly ask for landmarks. He doesn't care that the club is on Main Street, just that it is around the corner from McDonald's! In the club, an auditory guest inquires about the Nautilus program—wanting to hear about it—only to have the visual salesperson say, "Better yet, let's go take a look at it, that way you can see it first hand." The problem is that seeing it is not going to be sufficient for the auditory person. That could potentially become a major barrier. Can people with such different views of what is important really establish rapport?

SUMMARY

1. Rapport, the foundation for good communication, is nothing but a feeling of commonality.

2. One of the fundamental differences between human beings is our communication style. There are three primary types of communicators: Visual, auditory and kinesthetic.

3. A visual person creates pictures in his mind. His speech patterns and body movements are fast. He uses words like *see*, *look* and *picture*.

4. An auditory person relies on words and sounds. His speech patterns and body movements are slower than that of the visual communicator. He uses words like *hear*, *listen* and *sounds*.

5. A kinesthetic person relies on feeling, emotions and tactile sensations. His speech patterns and body movements are much slower than either the visual or auditory communicator. He uses words like *feel*, *grasp*, and *solid*.

6. Although every person utilizes all three types of communication styles in their day-to-day life, each one of us tends to prefer one of the three types as our "primary mode."

EXERCISE

In the left hand column, list all of your friends and family—those you like and dislike. Then, in the right hand column, determine what their style of communication is and write it down. You may realize that part of your "dislike" of some people is due, in part, to the fact that you have different styles of communication.

FRIEND	STYLE
_____	_____
_____	_____
_____	_____
_____	_____
_____	_____
_____	_____
_____	_____

5

ESTABLISHING RAPPORT

> *The ability to establish rapport is one of the most important skills a person can have. To be a good performer or a good salesman, a good parent or a good friend, a good persuader or a good politician, what you really need is rapport, the ability to form a powerful common human bond and a relationship of responsiveness.*
>
> Anthony Robbins, Unlimited Power

Knowing about the different types of communicators; how would you go about establishing rapport with someone you had just met, but that does not seem to be like you? If you are like most people, you would probably start by politely asking questions about the other person in the hope that if you talk to this person long enough, you will come across something you have in common (a sport, a hobby, or some other mutual interest). In essence you are trying to find out how this person is "like you." If a connection is found, the rapport process begins. Think of a time where half way through the personal analysis you found some common bond with the guest. All of a sudden the guest's attitude towards you changed, he opened up, and the conversation became much more comfortable. **Remember, rapport is nothing but a feeling of commonality**.

Selling Fitness

Suppose, however, that you cannot establish any commonality. Suppose the conversation goes as follows:

You: Have you exercised in the past?

Guest: No.

You: Any recreational activities?

Guest: None to speak of.

You: Well, how long have you been considering a membership?

Guest: A few days.

You: What do you want to accomplish by exercising?

Guest: Oh, I don't know, it just seemed interesting.

You: Do you have any type of goal or benefit in mind?

Guest: No, I just thought I might like to try it.

With the conversation going nowhere and the discomfort level growing, you know this is going to be a quick tour. You think to yourself, "Why is he even here?" What happened? The conversation never found that common interest needed to create a feeling of rapport. It seems as if the guest is a thousand miles away and believe it or not; he is feeling just as uncomfortable as you! This type of scenario becomes a lose-lose situation for both of you. Then what do you do?

THE ELEMENTS OF COMMUNICATION

Although we have all been taught to establish rapport through verbal communication (i.e., questions), studies done at The University of Southern California and elsewhere found that there are actually three elements which affect the level of rapport you have with others: Words including interests and experiences shared through verbal communication; voice qualities including tempo, timbre, tone and volume at which you speak and; physiology, referring to facial expressions, gestures and postures. Added together these three elements, words, voice qualities, and physiology, constitute one hundred percent of the communication process.

Surprisingly the study found that words constitute only seven percent of the communication process. Just seven percent! That can be mind-boggling information for some people. By observing communication between parents and their offspring, it becomes obvious that the study is correct. Children babble noises and make statements that are incomprehensible to others—pure jumble—yet parents know exactly what the child is communicating. Parents understand because they are put in a position where they must interpret the child's tonality and physiology. However in everyday situations with others, when words do not bring about commonality process, it is unlikely that someone will have the time and patience to observe the other ninety-three percent of the communication process. This results in a total lack of rapport.

Voice qualities constitute thirty-eight percent of the communication process. This means that the tempo, tone and volume of your voice is more than five times as important as the content of spoken words. A child who hears his mother rattle off his full, legal name is a certain tone of voice, knows immediately that she means business! Admittedly, conversation would be terribly boring without the elements of voice qualities—just remember all the classes you slept through in school. Remember the earlier examples of interactions between people with different primary modes of communication and how each felt about the other. The visual was annoyed at the soft-spoken kinesthetic and unfairly labeled him as insecure and unmotivated just by the way he talked. Conversely, the kinesthetic found the visual to be loud, obnoxious, and unbearable, labeling him as a con-artist and hyperac-

THE ELEMENTS OF COMMUNICATION

WORDS: = 7%
- ✓ Common experience
- ✓ Similar content
- ✓ Key words

VOICE QUALITIES: = 38%
- ✓ Tempo
- ✓ Timbre
- ✓ Volume
- ✓ Tone
- ✓ Pace

PHYSIOLOGY: = 55%
- ✓ Position
- ✓ Posture
- ✓ Gestures
- ✓ Proximity
- ✓ Facial Expressions

                                                       100%

tive. In the example of the two people who did not find commonality with words, there is a good chance that different styles of voice qualities contributed to the lack of rapport. Although similar voice qualities may have increased commonality to some extent, in some cases something more is needed to establish rapport.

Physiology, as you may have already calculated, contributes a whopping fifty-five percent to the communication process and the level of rapport you have with others. The use of physiology in establishing rapport is a form of biofeedback. If someone moves

Establishing Rapport

really slow and you move fast, you think to yourself, "Gosh, I wish this person would hurry up." But when someone moves at the same pace as you, and makes the same hand gestures or facial expressions, you feel connected to them for no apparent reason. You do not consciously think to yourself, "Gee, he is moving at the same pace as I am and using similar gestures." The brain though, receives stimuli interpreting that person to be like you, and you begin to feel that bond of rapport. How many times have you found yourself with a close friend or significant other and simultaneously the two of you make a move for the same thing or react to something in the same way, stopped, looked at one other, and laughed? It does happen, particularly with people with whom you have a deep level of rapport. Many times after it happens and you go to make your next move, the same thing happens. The charade continues, almost like a dance, until one of you finally says "Wait a minute, I'll go this way and you go that way!"

The power of physiology in the communication process is perhaps best evident on the singles scene. You are attracted to a person across the room. You finally catch her eye and with just one look, you know whether you should continue to pursue her or not. One physiological response makes such a powerful statement!

<u>Obviously, the traditional method of creating rapport by asking questions puts only seven percent of the communication process into conscious use, leaving the other ninety-three percent to chance</u>. This creates interactions where you really like the person or you don't like him at all. What would happen to your ability to communicate with others if you could effectively use the other ninety-three percent of the communication process?

MATCHING AND MIRRORING

There is a process that taps into the ninety three percent of the communication process composed of voice qualities and physiology. It will help you build a deeper level of rapport with any

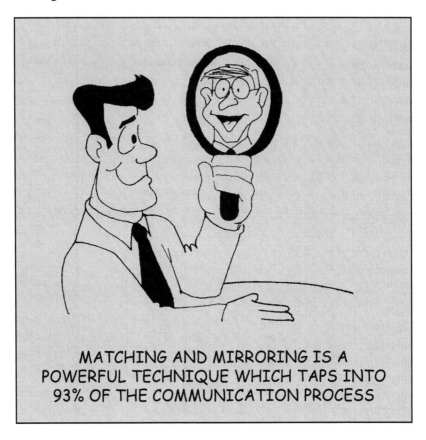

MATCHING AND MIRRORING IS A POWERFUL TECHNIQUE WHICH TAPS INTO 93% OF THE COMMUNICATION PROCESS

one. That process is called matching and mirroring and is a scientific approach to creating within other people a feeling of rapport and responsiveness. Remember, rapport is nothing but a feeling of commonality. <u>Therefore, matching and mirroring is the process by which you literally give the person with whom you are communicating the experience that there is commonality between the two of you</u>. This is done by matching and mirroring the various elements of their physiology and voice qualities.

Many people ask, "Is matching and mirroring the same as mimicking? Won't the other person recognize what is being done?" Obviously, if you sit back in your chair at the exact same moment he sits back or you go to scratch your head exactly when he does, or you cross your leg when he does, the other person is going to ask you if you have a problem that he should know about. **However, if you are subtle, the matching and mirroring process happens very naturally**. Whenever a large group of people are in a room, either sitting or standing, the groups of people conversing or congregating together are in similar physiological positions without any of them being aware of it. Smaller groups will all have their legs crossed in the same way, have their arms in the same position, or be leaning the same way in a chair. However, none of them will notice the similarity. It is never the people who stand, move their bodies, or eyes in the same way as you do that are noticed, it is always the people who are NOT like you. If you are still not sure, during a conversation, match the other person's body posture--subtly! It is very natural to change body posture during a conversation, particularly for the one making a statement or immediately after an individual is completing a statement. It is very rare, unless someone is making a point of not responding, for two people not to move and shift their bodies at all during conversation. So, go ahead, try subtly matching and mirroring. If you do it in a natural way others will have no clue. As you realize how effective matching and mirroring is in creating a deep level of rapport with anyone, you will become bolder at utilizing this skill. Even when you are not subtle, few people will "catch on" to what is being done.

BODY POSTURE

The first element in matching and mirroring physiology is body posture. <u>When you meet someone and begin a conversation and he is sitting straight up in his chair, you sit straight up in yours. If he is leaning back in his chair, you lean back in yours. Doing so will put both of you "on the same level," so to speak</u>. It is uncomfortable to talk to someone when one of you is sitting and the other is standing. After a period of time one of you will unconsciously change positions to match the other because it is more comfortable. What is done unconsciously can also be done consciously and the result will be the same—an increased sense of "comfort" for both people.

Selling Fitness

Many times when guests first come into the facility they appear defensive in both their attitude and their body posture. Sitting back in the chair with their arms crossed; focusing on people or things during the personal analysis. They are defensive because they know they are dealing with a "salesperson" and ultimately will be asked to make a purchase. <u>The mistake many salespeople make is that they try to *convert* the customer by showering him with an optimistic attitude and bubbly personality. Sometimes it works, but many times this type of behavior solidifies in the customer's mind that he is dealing with a salesperson.</u> You can avoid stirring up possible negative associations people have about salespeople by matching and mirroring the customer's body posture and attitude. What you will find is that once he realizes that you are not going to, "Isn't this great" him to death, he will drop his guard and begin to open up. Remember, people buy from friends, not salespeople!

MUSCULAR TENSION

As you become more and more adept at matching and mirroring body posture, you will want to match and mirror others' muscular tension and/or relaxation. Whereas body posture has to do with the position of the body, muscular tension has more to do with the physical manifestations of the emotional state, or mood, of a person at a particular time. For the most part, when in an excited or irritated state, the body is more tense. This is why when someone is very annoyed he is often described as being "uptight." One the other hand, someone in a relaxed or depressed mood, tends to be more loose, more placid. The state, or mood—hence the body tension—of each person in a conversation has a tremendous impact on the level of rapport that will be attained. If someone is really excited about something, spots a friend, and runs over to tell him the good news only to find their friend in a bad mood it affects their state of mind; they usually walk away wondering who put vinegar in his Wheaties this morning!

Imagine a visual person coming home at 9:30 or 10:00 every night, still wired from a busy day at work; to an auditory digital spouse who is actually in a low kinesthetic state from being a "couch potato". Having no knowledge of rapport skills this person bounces through the door, going ten thousand miles a minute, anxious to *see* their spouse: "Hi dear, I'm home, how was your day, did I get any calls, is there anything to eat?" If you have ever been jolted out of a deep sleep and recall how unappreciative you were of the person responsible, you can imagine how this person would feel—and what if it was happening every night of the week! Absolutely no rapport. Not understanding why their spouse is not as equally excited to *see* them home, this visual person attempts to cuddle up to their spouse but does not get the response they are *looking* for--their spouse is not interested. Both get angry. What eventually happens in this type of situation is the visual person's brain creates an association that says, "My spouse is not excited to *see* me, they must not want to be with me anymore," resulting in discouragement and their no longer attempting to cuddle-up because of the rejection previously experienced. That is powerful! How different could things be if this person utilized the skills of matching and mirroring? If the visual person would walk through the door, calmly, putting his emotional state and body postures into a kinesthetic mode, sit down on the couch, relaxed, and quietly say, "Hi, dear, how was your day?" Softly, "That's great, did I get any calls?" His spouse would light up like a lightbulb—a kinesthetic lightbulb— and be totally responsive and happy "to be" with them. It is that powerful.

FACIAL EXPRESSIONS

The next physiological element is facial expressions. Facial expressions can be fun. The next time you are at a party watch how two people talking about something with great intensity and rapport, will mirror one another's expressions totally unaware. Another couple will be talking and will at the exact same time begin laughing, meanwhile tilting their heads and bodies identically. Or, two people will be

65

talking about something very serious, and they both will tilt their heads to one side, slightly squint their eyes, press their lips together, and shake their heads ever so slightly. This is natural. When you are really involved with someone's conversation, you naturally go into the same emotional states, and both of you will express that state through facial expressions. <u>When you consciously match facial expression, it gives the other person a feeling of understanding and will create a better level of rapport with them</u>. Expressions tell others that you are involved and really listening to the conversation. Being "listened to" makes a person feel valued and important. Why is it then that so few people seem to listen to us? The reason is a lack of rapport with them! In selling, listening is one of the most important skills. Not only does it make the customer feel valued, but it is the key to understanding what customers really want from a membership— the emotional reasons behind the logical points they have expressed.

BREATHING

The final element of matching and mirroring physiology is breathing. Although it takes more of a conscious effort to match someone's breathing, doing so creates the strongest unconscious bond because breathing is biofeedback at the deepest level. When two people are breathing at the same pace, there is a certain calmness— a knowing that they are at the same level.

When someone is in a visual state, breathing is higher in his chest, an auditory state, in the middle of his chest and, a kinesthetic state, breathing comes from the lower abdominal. Mirroring someone's breathing will help you get closer to the state they are in and ultimately build deeper levels of rapport.

INTENT IS EVERYTHING

At this point some of you may be wondering if using matching and mirroring is manipulative. Well, if you go to another country and make

Establishing Rapport

a noble attempt to speak that language, is that manipulative? When you go to Japan and take off your shoes before entering a house, as is the Japanese custom, is that manipulative—or is it just courteous? Isn't it just good manners to change your style of communication to make others feel more comfortable? Communicating in your own way without regard to how others are relating to you, creates a lose-lose situation. Neither of you will feel particularly good about the interaction because you are being forced to take-in information which is being presented in a different "language." Sure, both of you may be speaking English, but both are not being forced to translate the information into your own style. What frequently happens in the process is frustration and miscommunication for both people. Start feeling good about all interactions with others and really learn how to connect with people by using the skills of matching and mirroring.

VOICE QUALITIES

The elements of voice qualities—pace, timbre, tone, and volume—will be quickly touched upon because by now you should understand how the matching and mirroring process works. Although all are important, perhaps two of the more influential elements of voice qualities are pace and volume. People have a tendency to label people according to the speed and volume at which they speak. People who talk more softly are labeled as insecure and quiet. People who talk very fast are just fast talking salespeople, and people who talk loudly are obnoxious. <u>If someone speaks slowly and you speak quickly you will not establish a lot of rapport with him. Slow down and speak at his pace</u>. Even if you have known someone all you life, and prior to knowing how to establish rapport you spoke fast and they spoke slowly, next time you talk to him, slow down, and you will be amazed at how much more comfortable your conversation will be—for both of you.

If you are the type of person who has always lived life at a fast, visual pace, you will be amazed at people's reactions to your new rapport skills. People whom you have known for years will tell you that you have calmed down. Some may be honest enough to tell you that you are a lot more bearable to be around—that you no longer emotionally exhaust them with the fast pace at which you interact. In addition, you will find that, because you are more easily connecting with people, and at a deeper level, you produce more energy in your relationship.

APPLY YOUR NEW SKILLS

The benefits of matching and mirroring can easily be applied to relationships with employers and co-workers. Have you ever worked for someone that, for no apparent reason, you just did not connect with. He is always polite and courteous and yet he seems distant. He is an auditory person and you are a visual person. He frequently expresses his concern about your "running around" to get things done. To him, you are not organized; he thinks that, "If you have to rush around, you must not have thought things through prior to starting the task." Is that true? Not necessarily, but that is how he perceives someone in a visual mode. Enter his world and you will be amazed at the response! If you are working for him, you will make you job much easier and establish much more rapport with him if you comply with his standards. What if your boss is visual and you are kinesthetic. He may perceive your lack of "visual" qualities as being unmotivated and unhappy with your job, the company, or worse, with him. That could potentially be more damaging than a boss who thinks you just run around too much! The important thing to recognize here is that matching and mirroring will allow you to communicate more effectively with others by creating deeper levels of rapport. What that means is having happier guests, selling more memberships, and getting a lot more referrals.

SUMMARY

1. Studies have found that there are three elements which affect the level of rapport you have with others: Words, voice qualities and physiology.

2. Words constitute only 7% of the communication process; voice qualities 38%, and; physiology 55%.

3. Matching and mirroring allows you to give the person you are communicating with the feeling that you are like him. Matching and mirroring taps into that 93% of the communication process that is non-verbal.

4. The elements you want to match and mirror are:

✓ Body posture
✓ Muscular tension
✓ Facial expressions
✓ Breathing
✓ Tonality
✓ Pace
✓ Volume

EXERCISE

This exercise requires you to have a partner. Another salesperson or a manager would be preferable.

1. Decide who is person A and who is person B. A will be the leader and B will be the follower.

2. Starting out slower and then picking up the pace, A, while seated, is to move into as many positions as is possible in a one minute period. Person B is to match and mirror them as closely as possible.

3. Next, switch it around, having person A match and mirror person B.

4. As you become comfortable with this matching and mirroring exercise, begin to match and mirror guests and members. Choose to use your skills with certain guests and not with others, taking note of how it affects the level of rapport you have with them.

6

MAKING THE TELEPHONE WORK FOR YOU

> *The telephone. Mention the word to some salespeople and they break into a sweat; to others, they drool. What is the difference between these two salespeople? Their income!*

Show me a salesperson that loves to work with the phone, and I will show you a salesperson that is more successful than his "phone-phobic" co-workers. In fact, if you are a retail membership salesperson, you should be spending anywhere from fifty to seventy percent of your time on the phone making contacts, scheduling appointments and following up.

USE YOUR SKILLS

In order to be effective and efficient with your phone time, you must use your communication skills while on the phone. Recalling the earlier discussion on the three elements of communication, you may remember that words account for only seven percent of your effectiveness, voice qualities for thirty-eight percent, and physiology for fifty-five percent. Because your physiology is not present when talking on the phone, how you use your voice qualities will account for eighty-five percent of the impact you have during a phone conversation. As a result, matching and mirroring the prospect's voice qualities is of the utmost importance. (Refer back to Chapter 5 for a refresher.)

Selling Fitness

In addition to using quality communication skills, persistence is a must. Every good salesperson knows that "no's" are not about him personally and do not necessarily mean that someone is not interested; sometimes a "no" just means that now is not the right time for the prospect. The persistent salesperson is willing to keep in contact with a prospect and ask for the appointment at a later date.

Of course, a good salesperson also knows that he must keep the customer's perspective in mind; a phone call is always an interruption. People are busy and their time is very valuable. Understandably, a prospect may resent the demand on his time at that moment. Asking the prospect, "Is this a good time" after you have introduced yourself, is the most courteous and professional thing to do. Doing this will prevent you from going into your presentation only to have the prospect cut you off or abruptly tell you, "No" not because he is not interested, but because it just was not a good time for him to talk.

As is the case with any sales work, you must discipline yourself when working on the phone. Commit to a reasonable block of time and stick with it. No excuses! Once you sit down to make calls, chain yourself to the phone. Make sure you have used the restroom, gotten a drink, pens, paper and anything else you may need. Let others know that you do not want to be disturbed for any reason.

Finally, create a worksheet allowing you to log the number of times you dialed the phone, how many prospects you spoke to, and the number of new appointments or re-books you set. Keeping track of these statistics is important for a couple of reasons. First, it can be a good indicator of areas you may be having problems with. Second, it can help prevent unwarranted frustration. Sometimes you can spend quality time on the phone and still not make appointments. This happens not by any fault of yours, but because you were unable to find prospects at home or were making most of your contacts with call-backs, which is always a lower percentage call.

THE INFORMATION CALL

As a retail membership salesperson, the information call is one phone task you must master. Unlike outgoing calls where you have time to prepare and get settled in, information calls come unannounced at any time throughout the day. In addition, the caller does not know who he is talking to and may be on the defensive because he knows he has been connected with a salesperson. These challenges aside, **the beauty of the information call is the fact that this individual has somehow been motivated enough to pick up the phone and call**. He has seriously engaged in a decision making process; one that requires him to gather more information than he already has, to enable him to decide whether a membership is ultimately going to mean pleasure or pain for him. It is your job-your duty-to make sure that the caller is educated as to what your facility can offer him in respect to his needs and wants. **In order to do that, the prospect must come into the club to tour the facility**. No ifs, ands or buts about it.

The fact is that no one can fairly make a major purchasing decision, such as a club membership, over the phone. Of course, from the prospect's perspective, there may be two or three facilities that he is considering. He may think that the best strategy is to call the clubs and weed out those that don't sound as if they will meet his needs. Although that sounds reasonable enough, you and I both know that there are many factors which should weigh into a decision that cannot be discovered over the phone. For instance, is the entire staff friendly and helpful? Do the members look happy and satisfied with the club? Is the club clean and well maintained? These are just a few of the many important factors that cannot be answered over the phone. Keeping all this in mind, let us take a look at a sample information call.

Selling Fitness

INFO CALL SCRIPT

1. Hi, may I help you?

2. My name is _____, who am I speaking with?

3. _____(Name)_____ how did you hear about the club?

4. Have you ever been into our club before?
    - If so, when?
    - Did you work out or just take a tour?
    - Did you enjoy your visit?
    - If not, why?
    - Was there something that you were looking for that we did not have?
    - Did someone go over membership with you?
    - If so, why didn't you enroll?

5. Are you presently working out? (If NO, go to #6)
    - If yes, what are you doing?
    - Where?
    - How many times a week?
    - How long have you stuck with the program?
    - Are you getting the results you want?
    - What specifically do you want from an exercise program that you're not getting now?

6. (If not working out now) Have you worked out in the past?
    - If yes, what did you do?
    - Where?
    - How many times a week?
    - How long did you stick with the program?
    - Were you getting the results you wanted?
    - Why did you stop?
    - What type of differences have you noticed in the way you feel?
    - What made you call us today?

Making The Telephone Work For You

7. (Name), that's great because we have a variety of programs here that are specifically geared for members who are looking for those very same things in a club. (Or fill in with a brief statement of information about the club that matches their needs.)

8. _____(Name)_____, what I would like to suggest, and I think you will agree, is that the best way for you to find out if the facilities will meet your needs is for you to come in and actually visit the club, how does that sound?

9. What times would you be using the facility, morning, afternoon or evening?

10. I have an opening this _____ or _____, which is best for you? (Here you are closing for the day of the week.)

11. I have times available at _____ or _____, which is best for you? (Here you are closing for the time slot.)

12. (Name), and _____ your last name?

13. And your home phone number? And work number?

14. When you come in for your visit, would you like to go through a sample workout or just take a tour?

15. When you get to the club, check in with the front desk and let them know you have an appointment with me, again my name is _____. (Slight pause) The visit will probably take around_____, so plan accordingly.

16. Do you know where we are located?

17. Someone from the club will be giving you a courtesy call the night before just to confirm and I ask only that if for some reason you are unable to make your appointment, please give me a call as soon as possible because I work by appointment only, okay?

Selling Fitness

18. Do you have a pen or pencil-I would like to give you my number here at the club.

19. I look forward to working with you this _____ at _____. Have a good day and I'll see you then.

UNDERSTANDING THE INFO CALL

Before we move on, let's take a minute to break-down each section of the info call so you can have a better understanding and appreciation for each and every question.

INTRODUCTION

As simple as it may sound, the introduction is one of the most important parts of the info call. Why? Because the introduction will set the tone for the rest of the call. Specifically, one of the two people-you or the caller-is going to take control of the conversation. If you answer the phone correctly, you will have a much greater chance of being the one who takes control. As you will come to find out, this is crucial. If you don't want to hang up the phone without an appointment, or perhaps feel as although you were just beaten up, you must obtain and maintain control of the conversation. This is done by asking questions.

The first question you want to ask the caller is, "How may I help you?" Now, even if you know the person on the other end of the phone is calling for information (because the receptionist put the call through), you still want to open the conversation by asking this question. Asking, "How may I help you?," tells the caller that you are there to help them, not just sell them. <u>Remember, most</u> <u>callers know they have been transferred to a "salesperson" and are probably feeling a little defensive to begin with. Start off on the right foot by asking this simple, courteous question.</u>

Making The Telephone Work For You

No matter what the caller replies ("I want to find out about your memberships, how much does it cost, do you have a pool, etc.), always follow-up immediately with the second question, "Great (or 'Yes we do'), my name is ____, who am I speaking with?" Notice, I do not divert from the info call script and go into a long dissertation about the memberships or our pool. I take back control by acknowledging the caller's question and then asking mine.

Finding out the caller's name is particularly important because being able to use someone's name during the conversation is a huge part of the rapport process. This is especially true over the phone where your physiology is not present. Although there will be instances where a caller won't answer you and will try and take back control of the conversation, 99% of the time this approach is effective allowing you to move into the pre-qualifying stage.

PRE-QUALIFY

The pre-qualifying stage is going to allow you to obtain information about the caller in relation to their knowledge about the club. The first question you need to ask is, "How did you hear about the club?" The answer to this question is important for a couple of reasons. First, you want to find out how the club's advertising dollars are working. Second, because "what" and "how" someone knows about the club has an impact on their perception of the club and the value it offers them.

Let's face it, someone who found out about your club from a summer special ad is going to have a different perspective and frame of mind than someone who was told about the club from a happy, long-term member. If the caller tells you they heard about the club from a summer special, there is a good chance that this individual is price conscious. They probably don't know much or anything about your club and will try and compare clubs by the price alone.

<u>If the caller tells you they heard about the club from a member-friend,</u>

Selling Fitness

 <u>you want to ask who that member is and if the two of them will be working out together</u>. This will give you an indication of where the caller is in their decision making process. If the caller hesitantly says, "Well, I'm not really sure yet," you can sense that they are still in the decision making process. If they say, "Yes, we plan on coming together after work," you know the caller is probably ready to buy.

The next qualifying question is, "Have you ever been into the club before?" If the caller has been in before you'll want to ask them some additional questions. For instance, how long ago was it that they visited the club? Who knows, you may have had major renovations since they were last in. You will want to know if they worked out or just took a tour? Did they enjoy their visit? If not, why? Was it something that the club was responsible for or something else? If it was the club you'll want to follow up by asking, "Gee, if you don't mind my asking, then what prompted you to give us a call again?" If they did enjoy their visit was there something they were looking for that we did not have at that time? Did someone go over membership information with him or her? If so, why was it that they did not enroll at that time?

In training seminars many new salespeople often say to me, "I can't believe that you are going to ask all these questions, won't that open you up to some possible negativity? My answer, "Maybe, but I would rather pre-qualify a prospect over the phone, making my job easier when they show up for the appointment."

A couple of other points should be noted here as well. First, it would be a rare call where you would ask all of the questions discussed in the previous scenario. You need to choose those that are most appropriate to the conversation. Second, it is the answers to these types of questions that are going to give you an understanding of what this caller has been exposed to, positive or negative, and give you an idea of where they are in their decision making process. This will also indicate how you should proceed with the call. Anxious to make an appointment, many salespeople don't

Making The Telephone Work For You

realize that spending some quality time with info-callers is what leads to a greater level of success. **Superficial info call conversations only result in a low show ratio**.

INFORMATION GATHERING

The next stage of the call is information gathering where you find out about the caller's exercise history. If the caller has not given you any indication that they are presently working out, you want to ask, "Are you working out now?" If the caller is working out now find out the details. Exactly what are they doing? How many times a week? How long have they been consistent with their program? Are they getting the results they want? (Keep in mind that even if they tell you they are, they probably would not be calling you if they were!) The final question you want to ask this caller, which is where all the prior questions have been leading us, is, "What is it that you want from a program or a facility that you are not getting now?"

If the caller is not presently working out, ask them, "Have you worked out in the past or done any recreational activities?" If so, get the details. What type of activity was it? How long ago was it? How many times a week did they participate? How long did they consistently stick with the program? Did they get the results they wanted? If not, what do they think were the reasons? If they did get the results they wanted, why did they stop? Finally, and most importantly, ask them if they have noticed any differences in how they feel. If they have already told you that they need to lose weight, ask, "Besides the weight gain, have you noticed any other differences in the way you feel?"

Can you see what this line of questioning is doing? Besides building rapport, by getting the caller to discuss what they have done in the past, you set it up so <u>they tell you</u> what they are unhappy with in terms of their level of fitness and health. This is important because the more someone discloses to you their fitness concerns, the greater the chances are of their making and showing up for an appointment.

Now, what do you do when a caller is not presently exercising and has never done so in the past? Simple, ask them, "When was the last time you felt good, or at least better about your physical well-being?" Although there are a few people who might tell you, "Never," most people will say things like high school or college. Follow up by asking them, "What were you doing then that you are not doing now?" The usual answer is, "Nothing in particular, I guess I was just more active. You know, walked places or rode my bike instead of always driving." This type of response gives you the perfect opportunity to have them affirm that there is a link between activity and feeling better by saying, "So, even that amount of activity had you feeling better?" Although this may seem like a subtle point, it allows you to gain some much needed rapport with the "non-exerciser" and bridge into the next question, "What types of changes in your physical well-being have you noticed since then?" or "How are you feeling now?"

Once you have found out about the caller's exercise history and where they are now in terms of their physical well-being, you now want to find out what the caller wants in the future (if they have not already told you). You do this by asking, "If you don't mind my asking, what specifically are you looking to accomplish with your health club membership?" This is an open ended question and for a good reason: <u>You never want to assume what someone wants from an exercise program. Let them tell you what their goals are</u>!

CLOSING

Once the caller has told you what they want from a health club membership, you want to peak their interest by letting them know that we can help them. For example, if the caller said they wanted to lose weight, you might say something like, "That's great because we have a variety of programs here to accomplish that weight loss and we have a lot of members who have successfully lost their weight and kept it off." In addition to peaking their interest, this state-

Making The Telephone Work For You

ment acts as a pre-closer. Once you have made a pre-closing statement, you must immediately move into closing for the appointment. If you don't, the caller will often try and take control of the conversation by asking you questions about the particular programs you mentioned.

How you close for the appointment is as follows: *"What I would like to suggest, and I think you would agree, is that the best way for you to find out about the club and see exactly what we have to offer you, is to come in for a no obligation tour. How does that sound?"* This statement has been perfected over the years and should be said verbatim. Once you have memorized it and can infuse some personality into the words, I guarantee that it will work.

WRAP-UP

Once the caller tells you that a visit sounds fine you are going to get some final information and then wrap-up the call administratively. First, decide on the day and time. This should always be done by using alternates of choice. "What hours will you be using the club, morning, afternoon or evening?" Then, "Which day would be better for you, Wednesday or Thursday?" Finally, "I have an opening at 9:30 or 10:30, which is better?" Always, always, always use alternates of choice!

What you never want to say to a caller is, "When would you like to come in?" People have hectic lifestyles with lots of places to go and things to do. If you ask them, "When would you like to come in," trying to sort through their schedule on the spot can be overwhelming and, for fear of sounding as though they don't know their own schedule, they end up saying, "I'll have to get back to you." What a way to ruin what was going to be a successful call. So, walk every caller through the appointment making process step-by-step, making it easy to set.

Selling Fitness

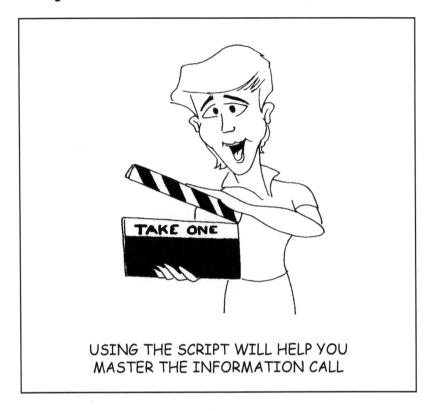

USING THE SCRIPT WILL HELP YOU MASTER THE INFORMATION CALL

Once you have set the date and time, ask for their last name and their phone number. Make sure they know how to get to the club, instruct them on how to check in with the front desk and tell them someone from the club will be calling the night before to confirm. Finally, make sure you request that if for any reason they are unable to make their appointment, or are even running late, that they give you a courtesy call because you work by appointment only.

TIME WELL SPENT

Now, some of you may be saying, "Wow, that is an awful long information call." If you use this script correctly and establish a good level of rapport with the caller, your average info call should take, at most, five minutes to complete. One of the biggest mistakes a salesperson can make is trying to close for the appoint-

Making The Telephone Work For You

ment too early, before the caller's needs and wants have been discovered. Some clubs even train their salespeople to go right for the appointment, something like this:

Caller: Hi, I was interested in getting some information and prices on your memberships.

Salesperson: *My name is Joe, who am I speaking with? And your last name? And your daytime phone number? Great, Casey, what I would like to do is set up a time for you to come in and tour the club. At that time you can go through a complimentary workout, if you would like, and I can answer all of your questions about membership. What times will you be using the club?*

I do not know about you, but I get bothered just thinking about a salesperson speaking like that to me. Image how the average caller feels! With no rapport at all, someone is asking you for your last name and phone number. The only reason that some clubs can stay in business with this approach is because their advertising dollars are bringing in such a large number of information calls that they can get away with booking a smaller percentage. In addition, those callers that do schedule for an appointment and show tend to be a much easier sale. Although large club chains are presently getting away with this, the consequences for the one or two-club operation will be devastating in the long run. It is hard enough to preserve a good, ethical, professional reputation; it takes years to try and overcome a bad reputation, particularly in smaller communities.

Take the time to establish rapport with every caller and you will not run the risk of being perceived as a business that does not care about its patrons.

EXCEPTION TO THE RULE

As is the case with many things in life, there is one exception to this information call format. This is the person who is experi-

83

enced with health clubs and has just recently moved to your area. If they call and say something to the effect that they want to come in to tour or try out the club, and you begin to ask them a lot of questions, they will get very aggravated. With this type of experienced caller, get their name and phone number, find out what their main interest is, and then book the appointment. You can ask questions when they get to the club. They know what they want and are ready to find out if your club will meet their needs.

WHY THE OBJECTIONS?

It would be nice if I could tell you, "Follow this script and all of the prospects that call will schedule an appointment." That is not going to happen. Some salespeople wonder why someone who is serious enough about starting an exercise program to make the call, does not want to take advantage of a free visit. Well, as serious as someone may be, people have reservations about making appointments. Remember, the prospect is calling you because he, most likely, is in the middle of his decision making process. He is hoping that you will be kind enough to provide him with all the information he thinks is necessary in order for him to decide whether or not he should take the next step (which is a visit)-but he is not that far along yet! He knows that visiting the club means he will have to talk with a salesperson who will ultimately ask him to buy. Therefore, you need to be prepared to deal with those callers who are going to object to your line of questioning, who are going to resist your offer for the free visit and who will try to take control of the conversation. Not being prepared for this type of caller results in your getting defensive and the caller either getting the information he wants without giving you any information, or hanging up angrily. Neither of which is any benefit to you or the club's advertising dollars. Let us take a look at some possibly difficult info call scenarios and see what can be done to turn the caller around and make the appointment.

BUT I JUST WANT THE PRICES!

I would estimate that seventy five percent of the people who call a club for information start the conversation by asking for the prices on memberships. Ironically, many of these people have no previous experience with a health club. They do not know what options are available with membership or what the prices should be. So why do so many people ask for prices? First, many people do not know what else to ask. They know they need more information but are not familiar enough with health clubs to ask for specifics. Second, most people are on a fixed budget. They are legitimately concerned about a membership being out of their price range-no matter how good it is supposed to be for them. Finally, as we discussed earlier, some people think that they are going to save themselves time and money by price shopping over the phone and then visiting only those that quote them the lowest prices.

The important thing to remember is to **not give prices over the phone**. Many salespeople think that giving out prices will please the caller and result in booking the appointment. It is a proven fact, though, that show ratios (the more important statistic) are lower in cases where price is given. If your present policy is to give out prices to callers who ask, (and you are NOT the least expensive club in town) change it! I guarantee that the time and efforts you spend role playing uncomfortable scenarios will more than pay for itself in increased show ratios and sales.

Because a majority of people asking for price do so for lack of anything else to ask, a simple re-direct is usually sufficient to get the info call back on track, putting you in the driver's seat:

Caller: Hi, I was wondering what your membership prices are?

Salesperson: *Great, my name is _____, who am I speaking with? And how did you hear about the club?*

Selling Fitness

Now you are right back on track with the info call script.

Does that mean that the caller won't ask about prices again? Not necessarily. Remember, some people are on budgets and price is a major concern to them. Therefore, the re-direct only temporarily gets him off the issue of price. Many times, either after you have offered him the complimentary visit or even after he has agreed to schedule an appointment, the caller will ask for prices again. **At this point it is important for you to acknowledge their concern**. Another re-direct will only come across as your being a "typical salesperson." I suggest saying something along these lines:

(Name), we have a variety of different memberships depending on what you want and the options you choose. When you come in for your complimentary visit, I can give you all of our membership information.

Then <u>immediately</u> ask the next question on the info call script so you can maintain control of the conversation.

Once again, although that statement works with many people, there are going to be callers who persist with their demands for pricing information. At this point you have a couple of options depending on your club's policy. If it is your policy NOT to give prices over the phone you can say the following:

(Name), again, we have a whole variety of programs and it depends on what you want and the options you choose. I can tell you that our memberships are both reasonable and competitive with the other facilities in the area. If you would be willing to spend just ten or fifteen minutes to come into the club, I can explain the club and all the different options we have available. What hours will you be using the club, morning, afternoon or evening?

If your club has a policy of giving ball park figures over the phone, you can use this statement effectively:

(Name), as I mentioned we have a variety of different programs depending on a number of factors, would a ball park figure help you out? (Wait for them to say, "Yes.") Our programs range from _____ to _____, is that about what you were looking to invest in a membership for yourself? Great, when you come into the club for your complimentary visit, if you like the club and think it might be the place for you, I can sit down with you and give you all the specific information about our programs. What hours will you be using the club, morning, afternoon or evening?

THE HOSTILE CALLER

Although the re-direct and/or the explaining why your club does not give prices over the phone works most of the time, at some point you will encounter The Hostile Caller. Why does an info caller get hostile? Ninety-nine percent of the time it is because you are not giving him prices over the phone. These callers are notorious for using the line, "Listen, I'm not coming in unless you first give me prices over the phone." The sad thing is that this tactic frequently gets the caller what he wants. The unseasoned salesperson gives in to this threat, not wanting to lose a potential sale. Learn how to handle the hostile caller and stick to the policy. Besides, if this caller is not willing to respect your policy and take a small amount of time to come in to the club, you need to seriously ask yourself, "Is this the kind of member we want?" So, the question is, how do you not give prices over the phone and deal with the hostile caller? There are a couple of ways. The first is by putting the entire price issue back into the caller's lap-nicely-by asking them:

"John, if you don't mind my asking, is price the only thing that you are concerned with (slight pause) or are you also concerned with the facilities, services, cleanliness, you know the things of that nature?

Selling Fitness

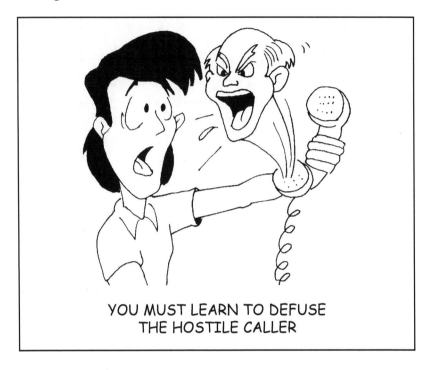

YOU MUST LEARN TO DEFUSE THE HOSTILE CALLER

If the caller says, "Yes, price is my only concern," (and your club is NOT the lowest price in town) you say:

(Name), then can I make a couple of suggestions. There are two other clubs that I think will best meet your needs concerning price. They are _____ and _____, are you familiar with them? They are the cheapest clubs around and, at the same time, I would highly encourage you to actually visit all of the clubs you are considering. Many of our members tell us that for just a few dollars more in terms of one's investment, you can get a lot more club, both in facilities and services. I would sure like the opportunity to show you our club and allow you to take advantage of our free, no obligation visit. What hours would you be working out, morning, afternoon or evening?

This is a powerful technique. When you recommend to someone that they go visit another club it usually boggles their mind. More importantly, it takes the sales pressure off. Remember part of their defensiveness and reluctance to come in is because they know you are a salesperson. <u>In addition to taking the pressure off, recommending other clubs will often create curiosity; a caller almost has to wonder what is it that your club offers that gives you the confidence to turn away potential business</u>. As you can see, this approach sets your club apart from others without bad mouthing the competition.

On the other hand, if the callers says, "No" to your " Is price your only concern" question, you want to say the following:

I'm curious, what else is important to you in a club? (If they do not quickly come back with an answer, offer them some suggestions. "How about friendliness of the staff? The actual facilities? Cleanliness? Certifications and qualifications?"

Once they give you feedback as to what is important to them in a club, follow up by saying:

Wouldn't you agree that those are all factors that you can't really see or find out over the phone? (Whether they agree or just remain silent, continue.) (Name), that is the very reason why we offer you a free, no obligation visit to the club. At that time, I will go over all of the membership information with you. What hours will you be using the club, morning, afternoon or evening?

This technique is very effective at this point in an info call because it really forces the caller to take responsibility for why they are being so demanding about prices.

With some callers you may try and use the "Is price your only concern" technique before you give them a ballpark figure. When this is the case and they continue to persist about prices, it is sometimes effective to follow up with the, "Would it help if I could give you a ballpark figure" technique. Remember though, the more you stay away from pricing information on the phone, the better chance you have of getting the caller to schedule and show up for an appointment.

Selling Fitness

THE REALLY HOSTILE CALLER

There are those few times when even the "Is price your only concern" strategy doesn't work and the caller gets even angrier. For those rare situations there are two statements that are very powerful and should be used only when <u>absolutely</u> necessary. They are as follows:

(Name), it is obvious that price is a big concern for you, and if you are concerned with price then I am sure you are also concerned with value. Sure, we could give out prices over the phone, but it is our opinion that the only way for you to fairly assess the value of a membership is to come in and find out what your dollars are buying. If you are willing to take fifteen minutes out of your schedule and come and visit the club, I will be more than happy to cover all of our membership information. If not, I can only say that I am sorry we will not have the opportunity to serve you.

OR:

(Name), I am not sure if you have had a bad experience with a health club before, but I can guarantee you that our reason for wanting you to come into the club for price information is not to try and coerce you into buying a membership here. We feel that in all fairness to you and us, one needs to visit our facility in order to make a fair assessment. If you are still that opposed to coming in for a free, no obligation visit, I can only say that I am sorry we will not have the opportunity to try and serve you.

Please take note: These last two are powerful, info call closing statements that should be used only in extreme situations. The reason that these are so powerful is that the first sentence in each statement makes the caller accept some responsibility for his hostile attitude. ("Obviously price is a big concern for *you*," "*You* must have had a bad experience.") In these cases where these state-

Making The Telephone Work For You

ments work, they do so because the caller accepts the responsibility and is put in a situation where his reputation-his ego-is on the line. Basically, you have dared him to visit the club. You have stopped defending your policy and have taken the offensive by saying, "Obviously you are not secure enough with yourself to come in and visit the club." Sometimes it works, sometimes it doesn't. One thing is sure, though, you have nothing to lose!

THE NON-COMMITTAL CALLER

The non-committal caller comes in many shapes and disguises: "I need to think about it," "I'll check my schedule and get back to you," "I need to talk to my spouse," and "The next couple of weeks are really busy for me," are just to name a few. Learning how to convert these non-committal callers into a more solid lead, though, is going to mean the difference between your making a good income and a great income. Remember, every person who actually comes into the club and meets with you has the potential to lead you to many more prospects-prospects that are generated from referrals, not info calls! Converting the non-committal caller into a scheduled appointment requires a gentle, non-threatening approach. If you try to push him into scheduling, you will only magnify his fears about coming in and being "sold." I suggest using the following four-step technique:

1. Align with him by saying that you either appreciate or understand what he has told you.

2. Smoothly bridge into the close by using the word "And," (instead of but which negates your alignment) followed by the phrase "What I would suggest."

3. Back up your suggestion by using the word "Because."

4. Ask for the appointment.
Here is an example of how the call might go:

Selling Fitness

Caller: Well, I will need to check with my spouse first.

Salesperson: *John, I can appreciate your wanting to check with your spouse, and what I would suggest is that we go ahead and schedule a tentative date, you double check it with your spouse, and then get back to me if there is a problem. The reason I say that is because I work by appointment only and sometimes my schedule gets pretty booked. This way, if the time is okay, I already have blocked off a time slot for you. The next two days that I have time available are Wednesday and Thursday, which is better for you?*

Always ask for the appointment. It will be a waste of your time and energy to use the rest of the technique if you are not going to ask for the appointment! Remember, the caller is still uncertain about what he wants to do next. He is not going to jump right into the conversation and say, "You know, you are right, I do need to come in and visit." Part of him wants to tell you, "No, I told you I need to check with my spouse." Another part of him, though, is thinking, "Gee, I already told this guy no once, and I guess the free visit is a reasonable offer." Use the alternative of choice, "Which is better for you" to close for the appointment and you will have a much greater level of success.

NEVER HANG UP EMPTY HANDED!

Lets us suppose that all of your efforts to get the caller to schedule an appointment have failed. At this point, many salespeople write the caller off: "Well, John, it has been nice talking with you. If you do decide to come into the club, please ask for me, again, my name is Joe." This type of short-sighted attitude can be very costly. Unfortunately, too many salespeople work only in the present moment-they are not thinking about cultivating sales for next month or next year. Top salespeople never let a caller get off the phone that easy. Before the non-committal caller hangs up the phone, you should be asking for his address and phone number. The conversation should go something like this:

Caller: No, I really don't want to schedule something unless I know that I can make it. I'll give you a call back when I know what my schedule is.

Salesperson: *Okay, John, that's fine. What I would like to do for you today though, is put you on our mailing list so that you will be informed of any upcoming membership specials. How does that sound? John, what is your last name? Address, city, zip? And, your daytime phone number? (Notice that the phone number is the last thing you ask for. Sometimes they give it, sometimes they don't.)*

BUILD A DATA BASE

If you always try not to hang up the phone empty handed, after a few months even the best salespeople will have a list of prospects that never made an appointment to come into the club. One of the best things you can do with these prospects is periodically send them something by e-mail. If your club has a data base management system that is integrated with e-mail that is great. If not, perhaps you can convince them to invest in a program like Constant Contact. However you manage it, in today's day and age using electronic media to prospect is necessary.

When possible it is a good practice to follow up by phone to ask, "did you get the e-mail?" This is a perfect lead-in to find out what was going on with that person in terms of their exercise goals.

This type of follow up to someone who never made it into the club sends a powerful message: "You are important to us and we want to keep you informed so that when you are ready to begin an exercise program you will consider our club."

Selling Fitness

Here are a few suggestions on how to keep an info-call data base working for you:

1. Make sure you date all entries as they come in.

2. Take good notes as to what this person wants and what his present situation is. Anything of a personal nature, even if it is just the names of his kids, can be referred to when you are speaking or corresponding with him at a later date. Believe me, a prospect will feel much more "listened to" if you remember these types of things.

3. Do not send e-mails promoting a membership special too often, maybe once every six months. You don't want to give him the impression that you always have some kind of offer. Instead, send him a club newsletter, monthly calendar or a flyer which invites him to an event the club is having. Once he has realized that you take the time to create long-term relationships-even with someone who has not bought a thing-he may be more comfortable coming into the club.

4. If your club has the capability, create a "field" that codes the prospects according to their level of interest, making it easier to do customized, mass e-mailings. Afterwards, make sure that you clean out dead leads and "Cannot Delivers" so you keep a clean list.

Building a data base from you telephone leads and keeping in touch with callers is another way to separate yourself from other salespeople and make more sales.

If you would like more information on how using e-technology at your club can increase your sales, please visit:

www.SmartClubMarketing.com

AUTHOR'S NOTE

With the current re-printing of this book, almost 20 years has passed since the first edition. Much has happened in the world of sales automation, hence follow up. Consider this; when this book was first printed a phone answering machine was a relatively new item and cell phones were the size of shoe boxes that only worked when plugged into your car charger.

Today practically everyone has a cell phone. Many people don't even have land lines in their homes. Caller ID lets the person on the other end of the phone know who is calling without having to answer the phone.

All of these circumstances make using the phone more challenging-- especially when it comes to contacting new prospects and following up with missed guests. Salespeople can make dozens of calls without physically speaking to someone. This is not an excuse for "not" doing phone work, but rather a reality that must be dealt with. As a salesperson you must learn to set goals, stay focused and most importantly be creative. Learn to leave fun, inspiring messages. Integrate e-mail into your phone work and bring automation to the workplace. Certainly using the phone has changed but no level of technology or automation can replace the personal connection that comes with a conversation.

CONFIRMING APPOINTMENTS

All too often salespeople think that an appointment made means an appointment that shows. Unfortunately, that is not how it happens. Although there is no guarantee that an appointment is going to show, one way to greatly increase your show ratio is to confirm appointments the night before they are scheduled to come in.

Selling Fitness

One approach is to have salespeople confirm their own appointments. The reasoning behind this approach is that the level of rapport already established between the salesperson and the scheduled appointment makes the call as comfortable and non-threatening as possible. Although this approach may be more comfortable for the appointment, it can pose problems for the salesperson. If an appointment is not serious or is in a procrastination mode, he will have an easier time rescheduling his appointment if he talks directly to the salesperson he scheduled with. In these cases, rapport works against the salesperson: He does not want to jeopardize a possible future sale and lets the appointment reschedule.

The approach I have found to be most effective is having **no one** confirm his or her own appointments. The best case scenario is to have a senior salesperson and the Sales and/or General Manager make the calls. The prospect will be less apt to try and reschedule, an additional amount of credibility and professionalism is created, and bogus appointments can be ferreted out. The call should go something like this;

Confirmer: *Hi, is _____ there?*

Appointment: Yes, this is he/she.

Confirmer:
- *(Name), this is _____ from _____, how are you tonight? (Wait for response)*

- *I am calling to confirm your appointment with _____ tomorrow at _____ and I wanted to go over a few things with you. (No pause at the end of this sentence.)*

- *First, do you have directions to the club?*

- *When you arrive at the club you will want to check in with the front desk and let them know you have an appointment with _____. As you know, he/she will take you through a brief*

Making The Telephone Work For You

personal analysis to find out what you want to accomplish on your exercise program. Next, he/she will bring you on a tour of the club and, if you want, will let you have a workout or sample some equipment so you can know exactly what the facility has to offer you.

☞ *At the end of your visit, if the club has met all your needs and you think you would like to continue, _____ will go over all the different memberships that we have available, okay?*
☞ *Finally, if for any reason you are unable to make your appointment, please give us a call because we work by appointment only. Do you have our phone number?*

☞ *We look forward to seeing you tomorrow at _____, have a good night.*

Confirming appointments is perhaps one of the most overlooked systems in clubs today. If your club experiences a low show ratio, beginning a system of confirming appointments the day before will increase the show ratio and the level of professionalism of the entire staff.

CALL-BACKS

Given the number of prospects calling and touring your club there is going to be a considerable amount of "warm leads" floating around your club. A "warm lead" is anyone who has shown an interest but has not yet enrolled. A previous guest, an appointment that no-showed, or maybe someone who participated in an open house event. Whatever the situation, this is someone who could be a potential member and should receive a "call-back" from the club. It is best that the person who initially spoke to him NOT be the one to make the call. Although this seems counter-intuitive, doing this allows the salesperson to ask questions that require the caller to get involved. Most of these questions come from the body of the information call or Personal Analysis. Therefore, if the person who initially spoke to the prospect were to ask those questions a second time, the caller would

Selling Fitness

sense that they were not "listened to" in the first place. This would not be good for rapport purposes.

There are four stages to the call-back; the introduction; re-creating interest, qualifying and closing for the appointment. The call should go something like this:

1. INTRODUCTION:

☛ *Hi, is (Name) there?*

☛ *(Name), this is _____ from _____, how are you today?*

☛ *I was going through our records and I noticed that you were a guest in the club on _____. Did you work out or just take a tour?*

2. RE-CREATE INTEREST:

☛ *If you don't mind my asking, what prompted you to come into the club?*

(Most likely he will give you one of three responses: "I was looking for a new club" (current exerciser), "I was interested in getting back into shape" (previous exerciser), or "I was considering getting started on an exercise program" (non-exerciser). Following the same format as the basic information call, you want to get the person to talk about what they are doing, what they did in the past, and what their fitness goals are now.)

☛ *Are you exercising now?*
    IF YES:
      ☛ *What?*
      ☛ *How many times a week?*
      ☛ *Where?*

- *How long have they been doing it?*
- *What is it they are looking for that they aren't getting now?*

IF NO: *Have they exercised regularly in the past?*
- *What?*
- *How long ago?*
- *Where?*
- *How many times a week?*
- *Were they consistent?*
- *Were they getting results?*
- *Why did they stop?*
- *What types of changes have they noticed since they stopped?*
- *What do they want to accomplish by starting a program now?*

3. QUALIFY:

- *How important is it for you to (get back into shape now?) or (start working out now?)*

- *Did you enjoy your visit at the club?*

- *Was there something you were looking for that the club did not have?*

- *It sounds like you enjoyed yourself and the club can meet your needs, did someone go over memberships with you?*

- *If they did, ask: What prevented you from getting started?*

4. CLOSE FOR AN APPOINTMENT: (If showing signs of interest)

In order to close for the appointment, use the "If . . . then" statement:

Selling Fitness

☞ *If I could show you how our fitness program could meet your needs, then would you be interested in getting started on a program here (or taking a closer look at what we have to offer?)*

Obviously, in order to make successful call-backs you need to be very comfortable with the information call format. You must be able to professionally probe and get the person to open-up and discuss their fitness needs. Your reward is a relatively easy sale, converting warm leads into happy members.

Remember, the telephone can be your biggest ally or your worst enemy. Make sure that you master your phone skills and do those things necessary to make it work for you!

SUMMARY

1. Because your physiology is not present when talking on the phone, voice qualities account for eighty-five percent of your communication. Use your matching and mirroring skills with your voice tone, tempo and volume!

2. Excellent salespeople are persistent and disciplined when working on the phone. Set aside a reasonable block of time every day, stick with it and create a worksheet to keep track of your numbers. In addition, you must remember that "no's" are not about you personally.

3. You must master the information call. Ask the appropriate questions and spend quality time with the caller so he knows that you have his best interests at heart.

4. A caller objects to scheduling an appointment because he is not sure he is ready to take the next step.

5. If a caller asks for prices more than once, acknowledge his concern and tell him why your club does not give prices over the phone or give him a range. Make sure you have memorized both statements.

6. If a caller gets hostile because you will not give him prices, keep your composure, reiterate your clubs policy and, once again, invite him in for the free, no obligation visit. If he continues to be obnoxious, at your discretion, you may want to use one of the two powerful closes I have given you.

7. With the non-committal caller, use the four-step technique: Align with them, bridge by saying, "And, what I would suggest," back up your statement with a, "Because . . ." and then ask for the appointment.

Selling Fitness

SUMMARY (cont.)

8. Make sure you never hang up the phone empty-handed. As a last resort, get the caller's name and address and start building a data base for future mailings.

9. Have a system for confirming the next days appointments- preferably where salespeople are not calling their own prospects or clients.

10. Use a call-back script to contact ALL warm leads.

EXERCISE

1. Make a copy of the info call in this chapter.

2. Take 10 or 15 minutes to familiarize yourself with it.

3. Have a co-worker role-play calling you to get information about the health club. Have them begin by being an "easy" caller and allowing you to set the appointment.

4. As you become comfortable with the easy caller, have them start giving you simple objections then becoming increasingly difficult as your skill level increases. Before you know it, you will be a master at defusing the hostile caller!

7
THE PERSONAL ANALYSIS

Up to now, you have been using basic rapport skills which help the customer feel comfortable with you on the phone and when you first meet him. What comes next is building a quality relationship with him, one where he not only likes you, but also trusts you enough to open up. The personal analysis is perhaps the most important tool to building such a relationship. The time spent going through a personal analysis allows you to sit down with the guest and find out about him, what he has done in the past in terms of exercise and what he wants now. It is here that you must use quality questions to probe for his emotional wants and needs. Remember that the prospect is driven to purchase by the emotions that your product or service is going to give him, not just by the product service itself.

THE GREETING

As simple as the task of greeting someone may sound, it is extremely important. You want to make the guest's first impression of you a positive one! Here are a couple of suggestions.

<u>First, if you are anxiously waiting for an appointment, do so at your desk or in the fitness area.</u> Many salespeople are so anxious to meet the guest that they wait for him behind the front desk. This is a mistake for two reasons: One, you are giving the impression that you have nothing better to do with your time; two, you have put yourself in a position where you can not observe the guest's movements in a discreet way, allowing you to assess his communication style.

Selling Fitness

 The most professional way to have a guest greeted into the club is as follows: Give the receptionist a list with the names of your scheduled guests for that day and the times they will be arriving. When the guest enters the club and asks for you, the receptionist can say, "*Are you John Smith?*" After he says, "Yes" with a puzzled, yet impressed look on his face, have the receptionist say, "*(Name) is expecting you. Go ahead and sign into the guest register and I will have (Name) paged.*" This is the type of first-class professional image you want to project to each and every one of your guests.

Next, once you have been paged to the front desk, try to take notice of the guest as soon as possible. Is he quietly waiting at the desk? Has he made his way past the desk to look around? Is he talking to someone? Does he look comfortable or out of place? Does he appear patient or impatient? You want to quickly gather as much sensory information as you possibly can so that by the time you have reached the desk you can match and mirror him. If, by the time you reach the desk, you are unsure about the mode he is in, or if the club is set up in a way where you do not have enough time to observe, be conservative. Moderately approach the guest, reach out your hand, and in an auditory tone and pace say "*John, my name is_____, welcome to _____, any problem finding us?*" Or, "*How are you doing today?*" You want to follow the greeting with a question that will get him to say something. That way you can tune into his voice qualities and have some additional time to assess his physiology.

A NECESSARY ALTERNATIVE?

At this point, some of you may be saying, "That ideal greeting is all well and good, but our front desk is a zoo at peak time and guests do not always get the service they demand, never mind this royal treatment." If this is the case in your club, and you feel you must wait for your guest behind the front desk in order to insure that he is getting a good first impression; make sure you have something constructive to do while you are waiting. That means no reading magazines, gabbing (non-work related conversations) with co-workers or members and never stand around doing nothing. As I mentioned earlier, you do not want to give your guest, or anyone else for that matter, the impression that you have nothing better to do with your time! Make use of this time by helping the receptionist check members in. This is a great way to get to know members names while at the same time you can be on the lookout for renewals and upgrades. <u>Working the front desk is also a great spot to give out guest passes and get referrals</u>. If your front desk has the luxury of more than one phone, you could make confirmation calls for the next days appointments. Whatever you decide to do, be professional!

GREETING WALK-INS

Greeting the walk-in guest is slightly different from guests with scheduled appointments. With a scheduled guest you have, at the very least, a basic level of rapport established. With walk-in guests you must start from square one.

Once you have been called to the front desk and find out there is a walk-in, check the guest register to find out their name. Next, approach the guest and introduce yourself, *"Hi (Name), my name is Casey, how may I help you?"*

Next, you want to run through a series of questions that will help you qualify this prospect while at the same time allowing you to zero in on his communication style.

"How did you find out about the club?" should be the first question asked since the medium that introduced them to the club will have an impact not only on the outcome, but on the sale process itself. Compare, for example, the guest who found out about the club from his neighbor who has a premium membership with a guest who found out about the club from a "summer special" advertisement in the local newspaper. Let's face it, these two people are walking in with very different frames of reference and expectations.

Selling Fitness

The next question, as a follow up to the first, is *"Have you ever been in before?"* If he has not, move ahead to the next question. If he has, you need to find out what his visit consisted of. How long ago was the visit? Was he in for just a tour or did he actually work out? Did he enjoy himself? Did he meet with a membership representative and go on a tour? If so, what prevented him from buying? Why is he back now? Asking all these questions is necessary. There is no need to waste your time or the guest's giving unnecessary or unwanted information.

Another question you will want to ask is, *"Are you interested in the membership for yourself or for someone else?"* I cannot tell you the number of times new membership representatives get through the entire personal analysis, tour and price presentation only to hear the guest say, "Oh, I'm not the one who is purchasing a membership, I am just getting information for _____." Unfortunately, there is nothing the representative can do at that point- he is left hanging there with the game-ball in the other court. Find out up-front who the membership is for and give your time accordingly.

A final but very important qualifying question that you need to ask is, *"Does your schedule allow you enough time for a complete tour today, it takes about twenty or so minutes?"* Obviously, you ask this question because you need time to establish rapport with a guest. To some walk-ins this makes sense and they willingly schedule a time to come back. Others, though, will tell you, "Oh, I don't need to go through a complete tour, I just want the prices." Of course, as is the case with an info-call, giving a guest prices without spending any time with him is pointless. You have no rapport and no knowledge about his needs and wants. Therefore, the first thing you want to do when a walk-in says he just wants prices is to explain to him that the different memberships you have are based on what areas of the club he will be using. As a result, he should, at the very least, take a quick tour through the club and let you know exactly what he will and will not be using. (If your club has just one membership, you want to align with them by saying "That's fine,"

The Personal Analysis

and then tell them that you will explain the memberships while you walk through the club.) Although these approaches do not work all the time, they are usually effective.

Once you get him on a tour-if you use your rapport skills-what often happens is the guest opens up and starts to talk about his situation and what he wants. Frequently, you learn that his reluctance was the result of a previously bad experience. After you have asked these basic qualifying questions, you can proceed just as you would with a scheduled appointment.

GIVING THE BRIEF OVERVIEW

Now that the greeting stage has been completed, your goal is to get the guest to sit down with you so you can begin the personal analysis. The best way to accomplish this and maintain rapport is to give him a brief overview of what his visit will consist of. As you begin to lead him away from the front desk or lobby area, say to him:

John, before we get started today, I just want to let you know exactly what your visit will entail. First, and most important, we are going to sit down and go over a few quick questions which will help me find out exactly what you want in an exercise program and facility. Next, we will go on a tour of the club and bring you through a sample workout or sample some equipment. Finally, if you enjoy yourself, find that the club meets your needs, and think you would like to become a member, we will go over all the different types of memberships that we have available. How does that sound?

As simple as this is, it can be very comforting for the guest. Many people become nervous and uncomfortable when they do not know what is expected of them. "Fear of the unknown" puts people on the defensive, especially when with a salesperson. Even if you covered this agenda on the initial phone contact and/or on the confirmation call, go over it one more time. I guarantee you, more times that not, unconsciously, the guest will appreciate this and become much more relaxed.

THE ART OF PREFRAMING

Before we go onto the next step in the personal analysis, I want to discuss a powerful language tool that can be used during the sales process. That tool is preframing. Preframing is the process by which, using the appropriate tone and words, you direct an individual's attention and focus. You "set the stage," so to speak. Perhaps using an example is the best way to explain.

Let us suppose that you and I have plans to go to a popular concert. We went through a lot of trouble to get the tickets and have been anxiously waiting for the show to come to town. The day has finally arrived and you receive a phone call from me in which I distressingly say, "Boy am I glad I caught you, we have a big problem tonight." As your brain processes that statement, what is going through your mind? Could be any number of problems, all of which lead you to the conclusion that were are not going to make it to the long-awaited concert. What if, on the other hand, you pick up the phone and I cheerfully say, "Hi, are you as psyched for tonight as I am? We are going to have such a good time. Listen, I have a bit of a challenge and I need your assistance." Now what is going through your mind? Once again, it could be any number of things, but it is probably not anything close to, "We are not going to make it to the concert."

These are both examples of preframing-how the choice of words and tonality of my voice preframed you to what is going to follow. By saying, "We have a problem," I am preframing you to think that what I am about to discuss is a problem. On the other hand, by saying, "We are going to have such a good time.... I have a bit of a challenge and I need your assistance," you are preframed to something completely different than a problem. How you preframe someone to a conversation will have a huge impact

The Personal Analysis

on their initial reaction. Think of how differently you react to these two words; a problem or a challenge. Most people hate having to deal with problems, but they are at least willing to deal with a challenge. Preframing sets the stage for the conversation that will follow.

What is interesting is that the information I was going to give you, which followed both of these preframe scenarios, is identical: "My car broke down this morning and since I was supposed to be the driver, we need to find alternative transportation." Although the example may seem silly, it is very realistic.

Unconsciously, we use preframing in all of our conversations. The question you must ask is "Are the preframes I use making others more or less receptive to the information that follows." Make sure it is the former, not the latter.

PREFRAMING THE PERSONAL ANALYSIS

How does preframing relate to the personal analysis? If you were to bring a guest over to your desk and say to him, "As I mentioned, we are going to start out by my asking you some questions that will give me an idea of what you want in a health club and exercise program," the reactions that you will get, verbally and nonverbally, will vary. Some guests will sit right down; some will reluctantly sit, thinking to themselves, "Why are you asking me questions, I'm the one who is here to check out the club." Others will come right out and say, "I don't need to sit down and talk, a tour will be sufficient."

Instead of taking your chances with how the guest will react, use a positive preframe:

(Name), one of the great things about our facility is that we take the time to get to know our guests. We like to explain our programs and to really find out what it is that you want out of a club. That way we can give you all pertinent information. We do this by using a personal analysis. The P/A is a series of questions

Selling Fitness

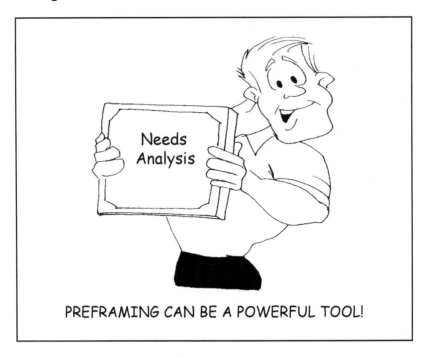

PREFRAMING CAN BE A POWERFUL TOOL!

about your exercise history and your current needs. Taking this short amount of time also allows you to find out more about our program here. (Place the personal analysis sheet in front of you, gesturing that you would like to start.) All right? (Saying alright? Rhetorically.)

After asking the guest "*alright*," wait for them to nod, say "Yes," or give you some sign for you to proceed. It is important to get the guests permission to respectfully ask questions about him and his health club needs and wants. In addition, his reaction will give you an indication of what type of person he is in terms of how he makes decisions.

For instance, if he pulls back and rolls his eyes, or gives some kind of verbal resistance, it is likely that he will be less willing to open up to you than someone who shows no reluctance to sit down and talk. That does not mean that he won't eventually open up. Once you have gotten his permission to probe and you use all your communication skills to remain in rapport with him, you will be amazed at how much

The Personal Analysis

he might share with you. Of course, this doesn't happen immediately. The questions you ask need to be presented in a way that is comfortable for the guest. Start with the basics and work into more detailed, personal questions.

USING A PERSONAL ANALYSIS FORM

Personal analysis, personal profile or needs analysis; whatever you choose to call it, <u>you must have a printed, professional looking form with some standard questions that you ask each guest during his visit</u>. I'm sure there are clubs not using a form and still selling memberships, but a form does a couple of very important things.

First, it projects an image of professionalism and gives you a certain level of credibility. Think about it, when you go to any other type of health-related office it is customary it fill out some kind of paperwork on your first visit.

Second, a questionnaire is an excellent sales tool during and after the guest's visit to the club. I don't care to recall the number of times that I, for whatever poor reason, brought a guest on a tour without using a personal analysis form and completely blanked and forgot his name. Too embarrassed to ask for it again I would muddle through the presentation avoiding any situations that would require me to use his name or introduce him to anyone; that definitely limited me. To make things worse, many times I would later find out that he had not filled out the guest register. This left me with no way of following up on a potential prospect!

<u>By using a form, you give yourself information to refer to during your tour and presentation. Later, the form is used as a valuable memory-jog for follow-up</u>.

EXERCISE HISTORY

More than half of the personal analysis is spent finding out what type of exercise programs the guest has previously participated in. The reason for this is twofold. First, questions about the guest's exercise history are probably the least threatening, making it a comfortable, yet appropriate place to start. Second, knowing a guest's past exercise history gives you information about, and insight into, his buying patterns. Let's take each one of the questions individually and find out what the information obtained can tell you, and how that can help you motivate the guest to buy.

The very first question on the personal analysis should be *"Are you presently exercising?"* You will find that the attitudes and beliefs of exercisers and non-exercisers are radically different.

THE EXERCISER

Someone who is presently exercising might come in with the attitude that he is disciplined enough to do things on his own but that he is interested in finding out what a health club is about. He may come in because he is bored with his program and ready to take it to the next level. He may be a member of another club where his membership is coming due and just wants to check out the competition. In order to get to the bottom of why he is visiting your club, you must ask questions.

Asking, *"What does your program consist of?"* is a good place to start. People are creatures of habit and prefer to stay within their comfort zone. What the guest has done before is an excellent indicator of what he will want to do in the future. You want to get the specifics of his program. *"How many times a week?" How long have you been exercising?"* And, *"Have you been consistent?"* These questions will give you an indication of how committed he is to his exercise regimen.

The Personal Analysis

"Are you getting the results you want?" is an important question, particularly if he answers no. The fact that he is not getting the results he wants with his current program is probably the reason for his visit. Furthermore, believing that becoming a member of your club will allow him to achieve the results he wants will be the factor that motivates him to enroll. If he says that he is getting the results he wants, follow up by asking, *"Then what brings you here today?"* Whatever his answer, keep in mind that if he was completely satisfied with his current situation, he probably would not be spending his valuable time checking out other options.

THE PREVIOUS EXERCISER

Someone who is not presently exercising usually comes into the club with a much less defensive attitude. He may come in noticeably out of shape, just feels out of shape or knows that he doesn't want to get out of shape. The common thread among all non-exercisers is that they have come to you needing to do something in terms of exercising. That specific something may or may not be your club, but the need is there. Questions are the key to finding out what he wants and why.

When a guest tells you that he is not presently exercising, you want to ask, *"Have you in the past?"* If he has, proceed with the same questions you asked of the exerciser, but in the past tense: *"What did you do?" "How many times a week?" "How long did you stick with it?" "Were you consistent?" "Did you get the results you wanted?"*

Now you want to get additional information. First, *"Why did you stop?"* This is a good question because most people have really lousy reasons for discontinuing an exercise program. Many times, a guest does not perceive his reasons as lousy until he tries to explain and justify himself. This verbalization process often gets the guest to realize that there is no "good" excuse for getting out of shape. Getting a guest to understand this makes the rest of your job a lot easier!

Selling Fitness

There is another benefit from asking a guest why he stopped exercising. When a guest gives you a reason that he perceives as legitimate (i.e. work schedule, kids, financial), you have created the ideal time to dispose of a possible future objection. For instance, if he says that it was his work schedule that caused him to stop exercising, you want to immediately feed that condition back to him in the form of a question: "*So your work schedule is not a problem anymore?*" If he says, "No," then he cannot use that objection later on.

If he says that his schedule could be a problem, you have the rest of the visit to get him to want to make the necessary adjustments in his schedule. In either case, you have moved the sale in the right direction. Make sure you use this technique for whatever reason he gives you for having stopped exercising.

Another great question to ask a former exerciser (which is not printed on the form) is, "*Since you stopped exercising, have you noticed any changes with your physical well-being?*" I don't care who the person is, if he has consistently exercised in the past and then stopped for any period of time, he is going to notice some undesirable changes. It may not be something as obvious as a weight gain. The changes may be something as subtle as getting out of breath when he goes up a staircase, but he will probably have noticed something. When he talks about undesirable changes he has noticed, you are getting him to sell himself.

If a previous exerciser tells you that he did not get the results he wanted from his past program, find out what he thinks were the reasons. "Was it the program itself?" "Was it the facility?" "Was it himself?" Whatever the reason(s), they will be of concern to him when choosing a new program.

THE NON-EXERCISER

As the public's awareness of "wellness" increases, health clubs are seeing more and more people who have never been involved in any structured, regular, exercise program walk through the

The Personal Analysis

doors considering membership. Although they may know that getting involved in a regular program is the best thing that they could do for themselves, because they have never done anything "structured" before, they often feel uncomfortable. You don't want the non-exerciser to feel completely overwhelmed and intimidated.

One way to avoid this is by asking him, "*Have you been involved in any recreational activities?*" When he can say, "Oh, I used to belong to a bowling league, or I gardened or I camped," as silly as it may sound, it makes him feel better about himself. It is important for you to recognize his activity: "*So you have been more active in the past.*" The point to all this is as follows: <u>In order to get someone to buy a membership he must feel that he is going to be better off exercising than not</u>. With previous exercisers it is easier; get him to discuss his condition now compared to when he was exercising. With a non-exerciser, recognizing his past recreational activity may help in getting him to realize the benefits of increased activity.

Another question that can help accomplish this is "*When was the last time that you were in good shape?*" Whatever his answer, ask, "*What were you doing then that you are not doing now?*" It might have been gym class or the raising of children. In most cases, it usually can be traced back to a time of being more active.

The bottom line, with the previous exerciser and the non-exerciser, is that you want all guests to consciously make a connection between activity and feeling better.

GOALS AND MOTIVATION

Upon completion of the past exercise history questions, you should have a lot of valuable information and a good level of rapport. Now the conversation can naturally and comfortably move in the direction of present fitness goals.

One important question is "*What is motivating you to get started on a program now?*" With guests who are very open to talking about themselves, they may have already told you what is motivating them without you even asking. You want the guest to know that you have been listening, but you don't want to assume anything. Feed his statement back to him: *"Earlier you said that the reason you wanted to get started on a program now is XYZ, is that correct?"* Wait for him to answer you and then follow up by asking, "Anything else." Try to get him to be as specific as possible. Saying that he wants to lose weight is not good enough. You must find out why he wants to lose weight (clothes tight, class reunion) and why that is important to him. Is it pain, pleasure or a combination of the two that is driving him?

Next, you want to ask about his goals. Specifically, what is it that he wants to accomplish? If he wants to lose weight, how much? If he wants to put on muscle mass, how big does he want to get? If he wants to tone and firm, where? The more he discusses his goals, the more he convinces himself that he needs an exercise program.

Once you have gotten clear on the guest's goals, you need to ask him, *"How important is it for you to attain these goals?"* Some salespeople feel awkward asking a guest this straightforward type of question. If that is the case with you, I suggest adding the statement, "If you don't mind my asking," to the beginning of the question. Whichever way, make sure you ask the question. The answer provides you with more valuable information. First, you get to hear from the guest how serious he is-or, at least how much seriousness he is willing to admit to. Second, the question will sometimes reveal a possible objection. For instance, he may say, "Oh, I think it is very important that I get in shape," and then add, "But it needs to fit into my budget," or, "I just need to decide on what type of facility to join." The more he says, positive or negative, the better. This is an information gathering activity. The more you know about his needs, wants and fears, the better prepared you will be to give him a tour and presentation that is specifically designed for him.

The Personal Analysis

The next question to ask is, *"Do you have a time-frame in mind?"* Meaning, in what period of time does he expect to attain his fitness goals? His answer gives you another indicator of how serious he is. It is also an indicator of how realistic he is. For instance, if he says that he wants to lose twenty pounds in six weeks, you may want to question his commitment to long-term fitness.

The last question, in terms of goals, is *"On a scale of 1-10, 10 being the greatest, how important is it for you to get started now?"* Note: This question is different from the, *"How important is it for you to attain these goals"* question, because the word now qualifies the urgency. A guest may say that getting in shape is very important to him but that does not necessarily mean that he is ready to get started now.

In addition to giving you a measurable qualifier as to the guest's level of urgency, asking the, "On a scale of 1-10" question gives you an opportunity to ask a follow-up question of those guests who give you a number less than 7. Looking at them with a somewhat surprised expression you say, *"Really? If you don't mind me asking, why so low?"* or, *"What is it going to take to get it up to an 8 or 9?"* His answer will further educate you as to his needs, wants and fears.

Of course, even if a guest tells you that he is a 10, it does not mean that he is going to buy. However, it does indicate that in his mind, he is committed to starting a program. "Which program and/or facility?" is the question that needs to be answered.

In an effort to answer the question, "Which program and/or facility is this guest going to join?" the last question in the Goals and Motivation section is, *"What made you choose us?"* Once again, although his answering this question by no means insures his enrollment, it does get him to answer in the past tense, and if he already has made the decision. Be prepared; there will be a certain percentage of the population that will tell you, "I have not chosen you yet." Do not get alarmed, this is all part of a control game for him. He wants you to know that he is in the driver's seat. Play by his rules. Look at him with a friendly smile and say, *"Well, what made you decide to choose our club as one of those you are considering?"* Approaching it this way allows him to feel in control, while getting an answer to your question.

Remember, though, that you will now have to do some probing during the tour and presentation to find out what other clubs he is considering and what factors will weigh into his decision.

HEALTH HISTORY

This last section of the personal analysis should be very brief. I want to make it clear that this section is not designed to replace the extensive Health History questionnaire the fitness staff uses prior to designing a guest's workout. The purpose of this section is to find out, up-front, if this guest has a medical condition that would require him to get a doctor's permission before enrolling. This way, instead of having a medical objection dropped on you like a bomb at the close for the sale, you will be able to customize your entire presentation around the guest's situation. *"When was your last physical exam?"* "Are you taking any medications?" "Do you have any previous injuries that may restrict your program?" And, "Are there any other restrictions we should know of?" All these questions should provide you with the necessary information.

AVOID THE PITFALL

In the selling of health club memberships one of the most gratifying parts of the sale (aside from making it) is having the personal analysis section go smoothly. Ironically when that happens and the level of rapport is high you will be tempted to make one of the biggest mistakes; giving out information about the club during the personal analysis, instead of waiting until the tour. I appreciate your concern. You think that when you are laughing and carrying on with a guest like he was an old-time chum,

The Personal Analysis

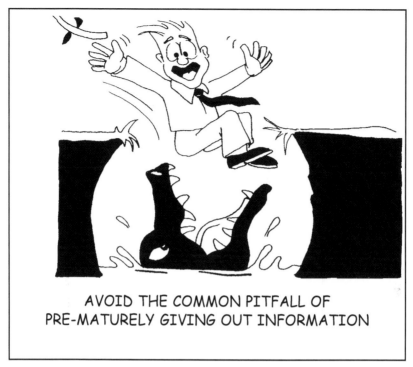

AVOID THE COMMON PITFALL OF PRE-MATURELY GIVING OUT INFORMATION

that you will break rapport with him if you don't answer his questions about the club when he asks them. Well, if you went into the doctor's office and he started to diagnose you before you had told him what was wrong wouldn't you wonder if he knew what he was doing? To me, that would be cause for a loss in rapport. In a way, you are a "Doctor of Fitness." Don't "diagnose" your patient or try and discuss a "treatment" until you have asked all the necessary questions.

SAMPLE PERSONAL ANALYSIS

Name: Date: Source:

Are you presently exercising?
If yes: What type of exercise?
         How many times a week?
         How long have you been doing it?
         Have you been consistent?
         Are you getting the results you want?
         If yes, what brings you here today?
         If not, describe the inadequacies of your current program?

If no: Have you been involved in any past, structured exercise program?
         What was it?
         How long ago?
         How many times a week?
         How many weeks/months/years did you stick with it?
         Did you get the results you wanted?
                  If yes, why did you stop?
                  If not, what would you have needed to make it a successful program?

If no structured program, any recreational activities?

What is motivating you to get started on a program now?
What are your goals?
How important is it for you to attain those goals?
Do you have a time frame in mind?
On a scale of 1-10, 10 being the most, how serious are you about getting started now?
What made you choose us?

HEALTH HISTORY

When was your last physical exam?
Are you taking any medications?
Do you have any previous injuries that may restrict your program?
Are there any other restrictions we should know of?

The Personal Analysis

SUMMARY

1. Because first impressions are very important, make sure that either the front desk receptionist, or yourself if necessary, is properly greeting every guest.

2. When greeting a walk-in, make sure that you qualify him before moving on to the personal analysis: How did he find out about the club? "Has he ever been in before? Is he interested in a membership for himself or someone else?" And, "Does his schedule allow him enough time for a complete tour?"

3. After the greeting is complete, give the guest a brief overview of what his visit will consist of.

4. Preframe the guest positively to the personal analysis.

5. Even if you have to have a copy of the sample personal analysis produced at your local print shop on nice paper, make sure that you are using a form which asks many or all of the same questions that this chapter covers. Remember you want to project an image of professionalism while at the same time having a tool that makes the process of selling easier for you.

6. When working with guests, keep in mind that your interaction with someone who has previously exercised will be rather different from someone who has never exercised.

Selling Fitness

EXERCISE

1. If your club does not use a personal analysis form that asks a majority of the questions given on the sample provided in this chapter, make some copies of the sample.

2. Role-play the personal analysis with as many different co-workers as you can. For each, focus on: A) Using your matching & mirroring skills to initially establish rapport: B) Ask him questions and give feedback in a way that gets him to open-up and talk about himself, and: C) Uncover his true emotional wants. Remember that you may have to ask questions that are not on the personal analysis in order to uncover the emotions or feelings that he wants. For example, "And why is that important to you?" or "And (working out regularly) is important to you because....?"

8

THE TOUR

At this point in the sales process you know about the guest's past exercise history, his likes and dislikes. You know what his goals for the future are and what is motivating him. Finally, you know if he has any medical conditions that might require him to obtain a doctor's permission before enrolling. Now you need to customize the tour by taking all the guest's information, matching it up with the features of your club and then tying those features to the benefits that are most important to him. As you will learn, this is a continuous process done throughout the tour of the club.

THE TOUR ROUTE

Being a creature of habit you may fall into a pattern of always giving the same tour; starting at the same place, going on the same route, and even making the same comments and jokes. The tour becomes so natural that you go on automatic pilot. I'm sure some of you can give a tour while, at the same time thinking about who you need to follow up on. When you get to this point, where you can give the tour without even having to think, beware! <u>When on auto-pilot-even though you are not conscious of it-you will be more likely to disassociate yourself from the verbal and non-verbal interactions that are taking place between you and the guest</u>. Hence, you could miss hearing a subtle comment the guest makes or miss seeing a non-verbal reaction. In an effort to avoid this, while at the same time touring the guest in a way that is most pleasing for him, I suggest that before you start the tour you ask the guest what he wants:

John, as you will find out, our club has a lot to offer; would you like to see the entire club today or just those things that are of most interest to you?

Selling Fitness

Asking this question is very important. Suppose that in an attempt to give the membership more value, you bring the guest on a deluxe tour of the club. What if the guest has no interest in many of the features you show him? He may not stop you from showing him everything, but he may very well resent it. You want the tour to help increase your level of rapport, not decrease it!

Whether he wants to see the entire club or not, the first place you want to bring the guest is to the area that is of most interest to him. With a guest who said he wanted to see the entire club, this means that enroute to your first stop, you will probably have to pass other areas of the club. The temptation here is to explain each area as you pass through from start to finish. I strongly advise you not to give a tour like that. Let me explain by way of example.

Let us say that you are in the market for a new automobile. Being the safety conscious person that you are, the most important thing to you is that the car comes with dual air bags (giving you a feeling of security). You go to a dealership and spot a car that you like. A salesperson senses your interest, approaches you and begins telling you about all the features this "great" automobile has to offer. While he carries on about fuel injection systems, the one question that is still racing through your brain is, "Does it have dual air bags?" Until the question about dual air bags has been satisfactorily answered, you could care less about all the other features. But once you know that it has what you want, then all the other features may start to play a part in your final decision.

The same is true in the selling of health club memberships. Before the guest can focus on or appreciate anything else your club has to offer him, he must first know that it can give him what he wants. Therefore, the first place you take him to is the area that is going to give him what he wants most.

MOVE AT HIS PACE

Add to the law of familiarity the fact that most salespeople are visual communicators and what you get is a very fast paced tour. Too often we forget that this may be a guest's first visit into our club, or any health club. Although we are accustomed to the environment there is a lot going on simultaneously in a club. This can cause sensory overload for many guests. Therefore, it is important that you tour the guest at his own pace. If he slows down to take a better look at something, slow down with him. I am not however, telling you to stop and give explanations. In fact, if the guest does not initiate a conversation, saying nothing or very little on your way to the first stop of the tour, can be the best thing to do. This gives the guest a chance to take everything in, get a feel for the club and maybe even find something of interest that he had not thought of before.

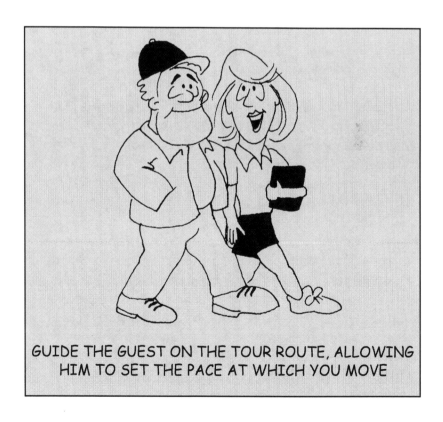

GUIDE THE GUEST ON THE TOUR ROUTE, ALLOWING HIM TO SET THE PACE AT WHICH YOU MOVE

USING A FEATURE-BENEFIT-FEEDBACK SYSTEM

You finally have the guest right where you want him-out into the excitement of the club and at the area of most interest to him. This should be the easy part of the sale, right? Unfortunately, although it should be the easy part of the sale, it is often the very area where the sale is lost. <u>The reason for this is that too many salespeople do not tie the features of the club into the benefits the guest wishes to attain, nor do they get feedback from the guest.</u>

Mr. Jones visits the club. During the probing process it was discovered that he wants to get in shape because he cannot keep up with his son when playing ball. Not only is he afraid of having a heart attack at forty-five years of age, but his sense of pride and how his son will remember him is a concern. The big challenge though, is his schedule. He is in a high stress job that demands a lot of hours. His time is valuable. The last place he joined had limited hours and classes. The mistake many salespeople make is giving Mr. Jones a tour that sounds something like this:

Mr. Jones, this is one of the areas that you expressed the most interest in, our cardiovascular room. As you can see, we have many different types of bicycles, stepping machines, rowers and treadmills. More than forty machines in all. Over here is the aerobics room that you asked about. We have over ten different types of classes that go on throughout the day and night.

The biggest problem with this type of tour is that it only points out the features of the club. Remember, the guest is not buying the features of the club, he is buying the emotional benefits he will receive from those features. Because he already has so much information to take-in and process, you cannot assume that he will make the connection between features and benefits on his own. **Therefore, you must verbally tie the features directly to the benefits which he wants**. Let's take a look at how you can take a generic feature of the club and turn it into an emotional benefit for Mr. Jones:

The Tour

Mr. Jones, our class schedule is one of the best because we have ten different types of classes that are offered frequently throughout the day. What that means to you is having the flexibility to come in at any time and get into a good class without wasting any time. And that means that you'll be on your way to feeling better about yourself, your physical well-being and your appearance. In your opinion, does the schedule offer enough classes for you? (Or, is the variety factor something that is going to be a plus for you?)

Notice that there is a big difference between this example and the earlier one. You are not just bringing Mr. Jones through the club saying we have this, that and all these other wonderful things. **You are getting him to consciously as well as verbally to say "Yes, that is good", "Yes, that will work for me."** Yes, yes, yes, like a train on a track. If he says, "Yes" to all the things that you show him-because you have showed him how they fill his emotional need or desire, therefore the chances of him getting to the table and saying, "Yes" to the membership are greatly increased.

Another benefit to this system of touring is that the feedback questions serve as a series of small "test-closes." As you may already know, a test close is a question you ask the guest about a particular aspect of the club which, when answered, gives you an indication of whether or not the club is meeting his needs and wants. Test closes are not threatening because they do not ask the guest to make a commitment about buying just give his opinion about one particular benefit of the club. Therefore, you must get good at being able to discuss the features of your club while tying them into the emotional benefits the guest wants, then asking a follow-up question which will serve as a test close. The format is as follows:

1. Make the claim in respect to a feature of the club:
"Our schedule is great!"

2. Support the claim:
"because..." (number & variety of classes)

3. Tie the feature into the logical benefits to him:
"What that means to you is ...(having flexibility to get into good classes and not waste any time.)

4. Tie the feature into an emotional benefit he wants:
"And what that means to you....(is that you will feel better about yourself, your physical well-being and your appearance.)

5. Get feedback:
"In your opinion....", "Do you think...." Or "If you don't mind my asking...." (does the schedule offer enough classes?, or is the variety a plus for you?)

By using this system you will help the customer consciously realize that the club is going to meet his needs and desires. This ultimately means more sales for you. The exercise at the end of this chapter will give you a chance to practice this on paper.

TOO MUCH OF A GOOD THING?

Although you would be taking your chances touring a guest without using the Feature-Benefit-Feedback System, be careful not to over use the technique. I suggest using it two, at the most three, times at the areas of most interest to the guest. Any more than that and you are going to start sounding like a broken record and come across as a "pushy salesperson." Besides, you do not want to pull the customer's focus away from the most important selling points by bringing to his attention to the less important benefits.

PREFRAME COMMON OBJECTIONS

As you know, aside from cultivating rapport, conversation made and questions asked during the personal analysis and tour are designed to ferret out any possible objections the guest may have. Of course, the earlier you know about an objection, the more time you have to try and overcome it. There is no denying that

The Tour

when you are at the close and hear an objection for the first time, you are at a disadvantage. The guest is now in the driver's seat. You are finished with the presentation and he can get up and leave at his own convenience. Therefore it is in your best interest to actually mention-by way of preframe-any or all objections that you frequently hear, before the guest brings them up.

For example, say that your club is a full-service facility with membership costs higher than your competitors. Over fifty percent of the time a guest will bring this up as an objection at the close. With these two facts in mind you need to preframe the price in a way that gets the guest to focus on the higher cost in a positive light. Let's say that during the tour the guest makes a comment about quality being important to him. This gives you an opportunity to preframe the price objection:

I'm glad you mention quality as being important to you. You would be amazed at the number of people who come into a full-service facility like ours thinking that they are going to get one of those $19 a month memberships that you see advertised on television. Of course, what they have not stopped to think about is that at those types of places you get $19 a month worth of service and facility. Let's face it, we get what we pay for. Sure, our facility costs more than some of our competitors, but as a result, you get a clean, well maintained facility and we get a more mature, responsible customer, who appreciates all that we offer.

Now the guest is focusing on the benefits of a more expensive membership. When you get to the price presentation, not only is he prepared for a higher cost, he may have already justified it with your comments.

If you have a lot of competition in the area, you will probably want to come up with a preframe for the, "I'm shopping around" objection. Let's say that during the tour you pass a member who had shopped all of your competitors before enrolling. When you pass by him you say, "Hi, Larry," then as you continue through the club you turn to the guest and say:

Selling Fitness

Larry is a trip. He came over here about seven months ago and put me through the wringer. He refused to enroll on his first visit because he had only checked out one other club in the area. He went to every club before he came back two weeks later to enroll. He was kind of mad at me because I wouldn't give him the gym bag that new members get if they enroll on their first visit, but he loves us anyway. I guess some people just have to see for themselves that our club has the best facilities and services around.

Although this preframe takes a different approach than the one on price, it can be effective because the guest hears, by way of story, that others looked around and came back to your club. If shopping around is not something that the guest really enjoys (some like the process, others despise it, many are in between), then the preframe may be enough for them to forego shopping around themselves.

With a guest who has never been a member of a club before or who told you that he had a bad experience, you may want to mention your club's Money Back Guarantee (if you have one). Although mentioning your Money Back Guarantee does not preframe any specific objection, it could make any number of concerns the customer may have seem like less of an issue. Halfway through the tour while walking between club features you can turn to the guest and say:

One of the additional features of our club that most people aren't aware of is the fact that we offer every member a 100% Money Back Guarantee. Meaning that, after 30 days, if you are not completely satisfied with the club we will give you all of your money back. That is how much we believe in our product and services. John, is having that guarantee something that is important to you?

Please note: The Money Back Guarantee should be discussed as something which gives the member peace of mind regarding his investment. It <u>should not</u> be used as a closing tool! If you

The Tour

find yourself trying to convince the guest to become a member by saying, "Hey, if you don't like it you can get your money back," it is probably because you have not spent enough time using the feature-benefit-feedback system.

Using a preframe in the tour may save time in the long run. This is not to say that no one will bring up an objection after you have preframed it, but it should reduce the number of occurrences or at least make overcoming the objection that much easier. <u>What you need to do now is write down the top three or four objections you get most often. Think about all of the possible preframes that might be effective. Write them down and then role-play using them.</u>

INTERACTIVE INFORMATION

Another thing you will want to do during the tour is give what I call interactive information. That is, information which puts the guest into a situation where he has to think as if he is already a member. For example, as you and the guest pass the front desk you will want to casually say:

John, as you may have noticed, for security reasons the front desk stops everyone coming into the club. Therefore, every time you come in for a workout you will need to bring your membership card with you.

As you can tell, the way this sentence structure is set up, it assumes that John is already a member and will be coming in for a workout. As subtle as this is, giving interactive information provides you with another opportunity to get the guest fully associated to being a member. Another ideal opportunity to do this is in the fitness center when explaining to the guest how the program works:

John, the first time you come in to use the fitness center, a certified fitness coordinator will be working with you. He will bring you through a complete physical analysis, to determine your current level of fitness. Then he will design a program based around

Selling Fitness

your level and your specific goals. He will write everything down on an exercise chart just like this one. Every time you come into the club to go through your program you will come to the files, pull out your card, and then write down your workout for that day. This allows you to keep track of your progress and when you are ready for a new program, the fitness coordinator can see exactly what you have done.

Even with things as seemingly minor as towels and locker keys, if you give the guest information in an interactive way, he may be on his way to feeling as though he is already a member of the club.

As you develop your sales skills you can begin to "stack" a variety of techniques. For instance, after giving interactive information about the fitness center you can easily transition into a Feature-Benefit-Feedback Module. They are perfect compliments to one another. Can you see how all of these pieces are beginning to fit together!

PRICE DROPPING

Price dropping is exactly what it sounds like; when during the tour you "drop into" the conversation about a monthly dues figure. For instance, you may be halfway through the tour and have discussed with the guest how the fitness center works when you turn and casually say to him:

Now, John, from all that you have told me about what you will be using here at the club, the membership that you would want will be $49.00 a month; (slight pause) we'll go over all of that when we get back to the desk.

I am a firm believer that-*with certain guests*-dropping in the monthly dues information (or a range) during the tour can actually help the sale. As you become more experienced you will get a feel for which guests price dropping is most effective with, but here are some of the more common situations where you may want to price drop.

For starters, if you have explained to the guest that you will be going over prices and memberships after the tour and he still inquires about prices more than once during the personal analysis; this is a good indication that he is very concerned about cost. Price dropping is a good idea with this type of guest because his concern about price is probably preventing him from relaxing, enjoying the tour and, most importantly, really hearing what you have to say about benefits.

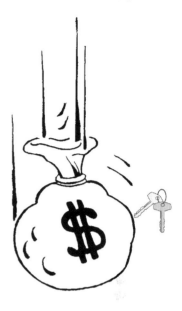

Another time to price drop is when you are working with a guest who has never been a member of a health club before. These guests have no reference experience as to the cost, and may be shocked when you get to the price presentation and hit them with monthly dues and joining fees at the same time. If you have price dropped, the guest will have had time to absorb and justify the cost of monthly dues, hopefully making the joining fee much less of an issue for them.

As odd as it may seem, I suggest you price drop with guests who appear to be an easy sale. That is, he is giving you every indication that he is going to buy ("Oh, that's great," "This is perfect," etc.). When you have this type of guest, throughout the personal analysis and the tour you think, "This is an easy sale" but sometimes, when you get to the price presentation, the guest does a one hundred and eighty degree turn and makes price a huge issue. With this type of guest I suggest that you not only price drop but that you follow it up with a tie-down. It would sound something like this:

Now, John, from all that you have told me about what you will be using here at the club, the membership that you would want will be $49.00 a month, is that about what you wanted to invest in a membership?

Selling Fitness

This way, if he says that it does fit his expectations, you will have less to deal with once you get to the price presentation.

As you will find, price dropping can help you make closing a sale easier. If, however, you are not comfortable with it, don't use it. Just know that with certain guests, not using price dropping may result in your having to work harder during the close.

MORE DIRECT TEST CLOSES

After using the feature-benefit-feedback system, you should have a good idea about which way the sale is leaning, but you want a more solid indicator. This can be accomplished by using one or two more direct test closes on your way back to the sales area. Here are three of my favorites:

1. *"Was there anything you wanted that you did not see?"*

2. *"John, studies show that those people who set up a schedule for themselves are much more likely to stick with their program, do you know which days you would come?"*

3. *"So, do you think this is going to be the club for you?"*
As you can tell, the third test close is more direct than the first two. Which test closes you decide to use will depend on your level of confidence as a salesperson. If you have spent quality time with the guest and have had positive feedback on minor test closes, you should not have any problems asking him if he thinks your club is for him. If he says he is "Not sure," it gives you the opportunity to find out why. If he says "Yes" then you get to your desk, go over memberships and move into the close.

SUMMARY

1. Before you start the tour, ask the guest if he wants to see the entire club or just those things that are of interest to him.

2. The first place you should be bringing the guest is to the place that is of most interest to him. Don't always go on the same tour route; vary it to meet the customer's wants.

3. Make sure that you tour the club at the guest's pace.

4. Use the feature-benefit feedback system two or three times when touring. That is: Make a claim in respect to a feature of the club; support the claim by using the word because; tie the claim into what that means to the guest emotionally and physically and get feedback. Remember that you want to get him to verbally acknowledge that those benefits are important to him.

5. Positively preframe common objections in an effort to dismiss objections before the guest has a chance to use them.

6. On the tour, get the guest as involved in the club as you can. Discuss the club in an interactive way, one that makes him feel as though he is already a member.

7. With guests who appear to be very concerned about price and sometimes with those that have no previous experience with the cost of health club memberships; price dropping can be an effective and painless way to introduce prices.

Selling Fitness

> ## SUMMARY (cont.)
>
> 8. On the way back to the sales area, you will want to use one or two more direct test closes, preparing the guest to move into the price presentation.

The Tour

See next page for exercise.

Selling Fitness

EXERCISE

In order for you to get good at using the Feature-Benefit-Feedback System, walk through the club and list the features that would be important to you as a potential prospect. Next, filling in the chart below, turn the features that are important to you into claims, give each claim support, then tie that into what that would mean to you emotionally and physically with respect to your goals.

Claim	Support
	(Because)
Our schedule is great.	Because we have 10 different types of classes and have at least 6 every day.

Benefit
(What that means to you is)

Feedback
(In your opinion, do you think . . .)

What that means to you is being able to get back into shape while at the same time having the convenience of a flexible schedule.

In your opinion, does this schedule offer you enough classes?

9

CLOSING & OVERCOMING OBJECTIONS

When I sat down to write this chapter, the first thing that popped into my head was, "Refer to chapters 1-8. End of chapter." Some of you may not find that as amusing as I did, but it makes a good point. Top salespeople put their efforts into establishing rapport, finding out what is really important to the guest and then showing him how the club can meet his needs and wants. They do not put their strength into one hundred and one power closes! If you have to close hard, you probably haven't done your job up front.

Although I do not believe in closing hard, I do believe that your time is just as valuable as the guest's. You are a professional who has spent a considerable amount of time to work with a guest. You deserve to know what his concerns are and where he is in the decision making process. Let's find out how you can do this and bring the sale to a close.

A FINAL QUESTION

You have brought the guest on a tour, have asked one or two more-direct test closes and are on your way back to the sales area. Once you and the guest are seated, you want to ask him this final question, *"Aside from membership affordability, John, do you have any other questions?"* If he has questions, answer them now. You do not want to finish with the price presentation, ask

Selling Fitness

for the sale and then have him start asking questions about the club. You can get sidetracked with questions and then you will have to find a way to ask for the sale again. This is no place to lose control of the conversation and the guest's focus. Make sure all questions, other than memberships are answered before going on to the price presentation.

PRESENT ALL MEMBERSHIPS

Although your price presentation is going to be geared around your club's membership structure, if your club has more than one membership, <u>I highly suggest that you show each guest all of your memberships-even when you are "positive" about which membership he would take. In general, the public is very suspect of salespeople</u>. It is almost as if they are just waiting for you to try and pull the wool over their eyes. Let's say that you only show the guest that membership you think he would be taking (it might even be a given). He then asks you, "Is that the only membership you have?" When you tell him, "Well, no, there are others but they wouldn't work for you" he is going to wonder what the other memberships are-even if he doesn't ask to see them. In addition, he may resent your assuming to know what he wants. The best approach to the price presentation is to say to the guest, *"John, let me go over all of the memberships that we have available,"* and then proceed. Start with the membership that you think is best for him and let him know that.

By including all the memberships into your presentation, you make it very clear to the guest what his options are. In addition you focus his attention on the negatives of the other memberships, rather than having him suspect that you are trying to hide a less expensive membership from him.

PRESENT IN STAGES

One of the biggest mistakes that salespeople are guilty of - as was I at one time-is presenting all of the information and then asking for the

Closing & Overcoming Objections

sale. Although this approach will work it is not the most effective. The reason is that by the time you get finished going over all of the memberships and their options; the guest may be in overload and not be able to process all of the information to make a choice. Not feeling confident that they are making the best choice the guest will go into the "I need to think about it" mode. **In order to avoid this I suggest that you present you memberships in stages.**

Let's suppose that you have two different memberships; a fitness only and a full-club. In addition to the different membership options you also have payment options; they can pay monthly or they can pay in full. On top of that if they decide to pay monthly they need to choose which type of electronic transfer they want to use; checking or credit card. If you were to lay out all of these options and then ask for the sale, it is understandable why the guest may want to take some time to think about it. Listen to how these options can be presented in stages making the decision that much easier for the guest. (Using a price sheet.)

John, we have two types of memberships here at the ABC Club; the fitness only and the full-club. The fitness only allows you to use everything in the fitness center only. So you can use the free-weights, the machines, cardiovascular area as well as take any of the aerobics classes. The initiation fee on this membership is $99.00 and the monthly investment is $42.00. From everything you have told me though, I think the full club membership is going to be best for you. (If that really is the case.)

The full-club membership gives you everything that the fitness only membership gives you, but it also includes use of the pool and the racquetball courts, which is what you want to play. In addition this membership gives you all of your court time free. The initiation fee is also $99.00 and the monthly investment is just ten dollars more, making it only $52.00 per month.

Selling Fitness

Once you have discussed both of the memberships, you want to immediately ask the guest, "**Which membership is going to be best for you?**" Once they tell you circle the membership type on the presentation sheet. This reinforces that the guest has made his choice and brings the first stage of the membership presentation to a close.

Next, you want to move into the payment option stage. It should sound something like this:

Now, John, there are two different ways in which you can get started on your program here. You can pay monthly, which is done electronically through a checking account or major credit card or depending on your financial situation, you can pay the membership in full and receive an extra month free onto the end of your program.

Again, as soon as you are finished describing the payment options ask the guest, *"***Which way is going to be best for you?***"*

By breaking the membership choices and payment options into two stages, you have not had to ask the guest for one big decision-you have just asked him for two much smaller decisions.

SHUT-UP!

Have you heard the expression, "There is a time to be heard and a time to remain silent?" Well, **after you have asked for the sale it's time to remain silent.** Too many salespeople babble on after the close. The reason of course, is that they are uncomfortable with the silence. I agree that it is uncomfortable, but that's life. I don't care if the guest sits there quietly for three, four or five minutes-do not be the one to break the silence. If the silence is making you that uncomfortable, find some papers to shuffle or even call the front desk to find out if you have any messages. Perhaps what my first manager used to say to me will drive the point home: "He who speaks first has bought it." Since you are not the one who needs to buy a membership, don't speak first!

Closing & Overcoming Objections

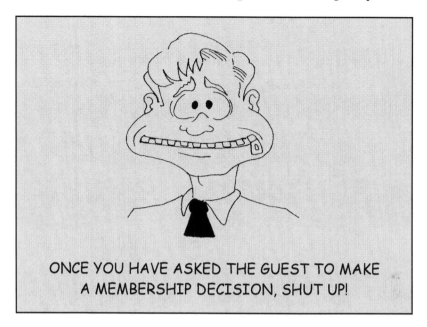

ONCE YOU HAVE ASKED THE GUEST TO MAKE A MEMBERSHIP DECISION, SHUT UP!

ASK FOR THE SALE

Once the guest has made his choices regarding membership type and payment option, you have to ask for the sale. Although it may seem silly for me to point this out, you would be amazed at the number of salespeople who, for whatever reason, don't do it. The reason, of course, is they feel funny asking for money. This is particularly true of new salespeople. I can assure you though, unless you ask, most people are not going to say to you "So, can I get started now?" If you have followed the steps for presenting in stages, the easiest way to ask for the sale is to not ask at all-just **assume the sale!** Remember, the guest has already told you that one of the memberships and one of the payment options are going to be best for them. All you have to say is, *"Great, let me go ahead and get the paperwork."* If they are ready to buy they won't flinch. If they are not, trust me, they will tell you.

If for some reason you feel uncomfortable assuming the sale, you can simply ask, *"Would you like to get started today?"* Personally, I do not think this approach is as effective as the assumptive close because it gives the guest a chance to easily say to you, "No, I don't want to get started." Believe it or not, many people <u>want you</u> to close them on a membership. They know they need to get started yet they can't seem to make the decision themselves. If you give them another opportunity to procrastinate you are doing them no service.

<u>Remember, though, the approach you use to close the sale is not the all-important. What is important is that you close</u>! If you don't close the sale, nine times out of ten the guest will say, "Thanks for the information," get up from the table and leave. At that point you are in no position to start asking for the sale.

WELCOME OBJECTIONS

Salesperson or not, no one like to be rejected. Even though you logically know that an objection is not about you personally, it can be hard for you to deal with them. You may think objections are these terrible obstacles which prevent you from making more sales. Nothing could be farther from the truth. Objections actually give you an opportunity to close the sale because in essence, the guest is saying, "I would buy, but there is this problem." Meaning, if you can find a solution to his objection then he will buy. Imagine if instead of giving you an objection a guest just said, "That is very interesting, thanks for the information," and got up to leave. You would feel pretty silly asking for the sale as they were walking away from you. So you see, an objection gives you an opportunity to engage in more conversation giving you another chance to show the customer how buying will give him pleasure, and how not buying will give him pain.

WHY OBJECTIONS?

Just for a moment, put yourself in the guest's shoes. You have just spent forty-five minutes with a very pleasant salesperson at this health club. There is no question that the facility is nice but, at the unconscious level your brain has not completely sorted out the

Closing & Overcoming Objections

potential pleasures and pains of the purchase. You just don't know what to do. The salesperson has asked you to make a decision and it has been dead silence since. You are starting to feel a bit uncomfortable and would really like to have some time to think things over; you know, weigh-out the pros and cons. This salesperson has been so nice to you though that you don't want to come right out and say, "I don't want to buy." What you decide to do is give the salesperson a "reasonable" objection in the hopes that he will let you leave and you can call them back with your decision.

Let's face it, we have all been in situations where someone asked us to buy their product or service and we did not want to make a decision right there. It could have been the kid selling cookies at your front door or the insurance agent asking you to buy a policy. By using an objection or two, you figured you could buy some time. With the kid selling cookies it might have been, "Let me make sure my wife didn't already buy some from her friend at work." With the insurance agent it might have been, "I really need to completely assess all my needs before I make a decision. Let me get back to you some time next week." Almost all objections are an attempt by the prospect to buy some time **because he is not sure that the pleasure of the membership will outweigh the pain of spending his money.**

Because we have all been there you should appreciate how the guest is feeling. At the same time, you need to keep in mind that when a guest leaves the facility, you no longer have an impact on what he is focusing on. Consequently, you need to work with him so both of you can better understand what the real issue is and try to find a solution. Although one cannot say, "This is the way you overcome a certain objection," let's take a look at some steps which can help you overcome objections. Remember though, every objection is unique and must be treated accordingly.

RELAX AND FEED IT BACK

Once a guest has given you an objection, the first thing you want to do is relax. Too many times the salesperson that has memorized closes will immediately respond to the guest's objection sometimes before he has even finished what he is saying. Make sure you do not do this. You want to take your time and find out what the guest's real concerns are. When he has clearly finished giving you his objection nicely feed it back to him in the form of a question and then be quiet. Many people use an initial objection as a smoke screen or just a way to procrastinate from making a decision right then and there. By putting the objection back in his lap, he will do one of three things. One, he will have to stick with his initial objection, "Yes, it is too expensive." Two, he will have to use another objection, "Well, it's really that I'm just not sure I will use it." Third, if he was just procrastinating, he may decide to buy.

ALIGN WITH HIM

After defending their objection, you may notice that some guests body language will become defensive, as if they are readying to defend their position. Therefore after a prospect has stood by his objection, the first thing you want to do is align with him. One way to effectively align with him is by using the "feel, felt, found" statements:

John, I can appreciate your feeling that the membership is too expensive. Many of our members felt the same way at first and you know what they found was....

By aligning with the prospect, you take the pressure off of him. He is relieved that you understand how he feels. In addition, he is pleasantly surprised that you are not trying to push him into buying. The result is your maintaining the highest possible level of rapport and getting the prospect off the defensive.

Closing & Overcoming Objections

Another benefit to using the "feel, felt, found" statement is that it uses third party stories. <u>Human beings are much more receptive to stories about other people because they can relate to them from a non-authoritative position</u>. You-as the salesperson-aren't telling them what to do; you are merely sharing with them the common experience of a guest who was just like them. Knowing that others have felt the same way also takes some of the sales pressure off the guest.

QUESTION IT

After you have aligned with the guest, you want to politely question him. *"John, I know you have reasons for saying that, do you mind if I ask what they are?"* When you question the guest he will start trying to justify himself. This often leads to his talking himself right out of the objection and into buying the membership.

ISOLATE THE OBJECTION

Once you have aligned with the prospect, you want to isolate his objection. If you are successful at overcoming one objection, you do not want him to reply with a, "Well, that really is not the problem, the real problem is _____." How you isolate an objection is by asking a "just suppose" frame. For example:

John, just suppose we could handle _____, in your opinion do you feel as though you would go ahead with the purchase?," or *"John, just suppose you did not have to discuss the purchase with your wife, would you want to go ahead with the purchase?*

You are asking them to make a commitment that says, "If we did not have this **one** obstacle to overcome, I would buy." Only until you have isolated the objection can you overcome it.

REFRAME

Once you have isolated the guest's objection, the next thing you need to do is "reframe" it. Just as an artist can place different frames around a picture to completely change it's look and how the viewer sees it, you can use a reframe to change the way a guest "sees" an objection. You actually get the guest to change what he is focusing on.

For example, let's say that the prospect's objection is that the initiation fee is too expensive. You could sit there all day and try and convince him that the initiation fee is not too expensive, but most likely, his belief will still be that it is too expensive. One reframe for this objection might be:

John, in spite of the cost of the initiation fee, isn't the real question how we can find a way to get you started so that you can start feeling better about your health?

The reframe takes his focus off of the prices and puts it back on the emotional and physical benefits he wants most as a result of having a membership. If the guest agrees with you that this is the issue, he is now committing to focus his attention on finding a solution.

CLOSE AGAIN

Now that you have the guest's focus back on the emotional and physical benefits he wants from the membership, you want to close again. There are a number of strategies you can use.

One way you could close again is by outweighing the objection. If the guest said that the program was "Too expensive," you would outweigh that by saying something like,

John, I know you want to feel better about yourself and I know that you are concerned about the cost, but isn't your health the more important of the two?

Closing & Overcoming Objections

Unless your membership is some exorbitant amount, there are very few people who would say that their health is not worth fifty to one hundred dollars a month!

A second way to close again is to turn-around the objection. If someone gave you the "I don't think I'll stick with it" objection, you could turn it around by saying, *"John, isn't that the very reason you need to get started?"* With the turn around objection it is very important that you offer no explanation for turning the objection around. You want to let the guest come to his own conclusions. By saying, "Isn't that the very reason you need to get started," you are asking his brain to come up with a reason why he should get started. If you try to offer support-in the form of your opinion-his brain is no longer searching for it's own answer. Instead, it is evaluating the legitimacy of your opinion, which most likely he will not completely agree with.

A third way to close again is to explain it. If the objection is that the membership is too expensive you explain why that is the case:

Yes, our membership here is more expensive that our competitors and, as I mentioned earlier, the reasons for that are_____, all features that will help you get what you want most.

A final way that you can close again is by "minimizing" the objection. If the objection is that the membership is too expensive, you first find out by how much the person thinks it is too expensive. Were they planning on spending $700.00 a year versus $850.00? If that is the case, you minimize it by saying:

So, that's $150.00 a year, which is about $12.00 a month, which comes our to less than fifty cents a day. John, are you going to let fifty cents a day get in the way of your feeling more self-confident and looking the way you really want to?

By minimizing the objection, you are able to effectively use contrast. Most people will not say that they are willing to sacrifice something as important as their health for fifty cents a day.

Selling Fitness

Once you have gotten some experience using these different closes you will learn how to mix elements of each one into new and powerful statements.

ESTABLISH A COURSE OF CONTACT

Of course, there will be those guests who decide not to make a purchase that day. When this happens, the most important thing that you can do is to establish a course of contact with them. This can be done one of two ways. First, if the guest has not used the club, you may want to invite them back for a sample workout. That conversation should go as follows:

John, it seems that you are serious about starting a regular exercise program and that our facility might be the right one for you. Let me ask you, if I were able to arrange it so you could come in and use the club for a day or two, just as if you were a new member, would that allow you to make a more educated decision?

If the guest says, "Yes," you will want to use alternates of choice to determine exactly what day(s) they will be using the club, and at what time. Once this is determined, fill out a guest pass so it reflects those times only. This way, you can make a note in your appointment book and be prepared to touch base with the guest when he is in the club.

If, however, the guest says, "No, I don't need to try out the club," your next step is to decide on a day that the two of you will talk. The conversation may go something like this:

That's fine John, obviously you know what you want in a club. Do you mind my asking, about how long will it be before you make a decision? A day, two days, a week?

Once the guest gives you a answer, continue with booking a course of contact:

Closing & Overcoming Objections

Great. Let's see, today is _____. So, if I don't hear back from you by _____, would it be okay if I gave you a call?

Once they say, "Yes," set an exact time:

What time of day would be better, morning, afternoon or evening? Okay, I have times available at _____ or _____, which is best for you?

Of course, this isn't to say that the guest will answer his phone at the designated time, he may not. <u>However, by having a specific time set, not only are you seen as more of a professional, but you have now gotten the guest's permission to follow up</u>!

It is imperative that you establish a line of communication with every guest before they leave the club. You do not want to be sitting by the phone wondering when a guest is going to call you back. Remember that you are a professional. If you have done your job right you have earned the right to be informed in a timely fashion.

COMMON OBJECTIONS

Although every individual's circumstances are unique, fitness salespeople have been hearing the same objections for the past twenty-five years. This section is designed to introduce you to the most common objections and give you sample scenarios of how they could be handled.

I NEED TO THINK ABOUT IT

"I need to think about it" is the most common objection you will hear. Most guests use it as a smoke screen to their real objection. Never, never, never let a prospect walk out of your club telling you that he needs to think about it. Once he leaves, you will probably never find out what the real objection is. Therefore, you will not be able to find a solution to his concerns. Here is one example of how

Selling Fitness

you can deal with this objection. Notice that instead of feeding back the "I need to think about it" objection, you try and qualify what part of the decision he needs to think about.

Guest: I need to think about it.

Salesperson: *That's fine, John, I can appreciate your needing to think about it. Making a commitment to exercise is an important decision. If you don't mind me asking, what part of your decision is it that you need to think about? Is it the club, the facilities. . . or could it be the investment?*

Once you have asked the question, be quiet! What will usually follow is the guest disclosing what the real objection is.

IT'S TOO EXPENSIVE

The first step in dealing with the "It's too expensive" objection is qualifying exactly what is too expensive-the initiation fee or the monthly dues.

Salesperson: *John, I can appreciate your feeling that the program is expensive. If you don't mind my asking what is it that you find expensive, the initiation fee or the monthly dues?*

If they say that it is the initiation fee that is too expensive, this is what you will want to say:

Salesperson: *So, the monthly amount is okay, it's just the initiation fee that you feel is too expensive?*

<u>Saying this accomplishes two things. First, it gets them to say "Yes" the monthly amount is okay, while at the same time it is isolating the initiation fee objection.</u>

Closing & Overcoming Objections

Next, question it:

Salesperson: *I know you have reasons for saying that, do you mind if I ask what they are?*

Guest: I just wasn't expecting to spend that much up front.

Now, isolate the objection:

Salesperson: *John, if the initiation was not an issue, in your opinion do you feel as if you would go ahead and get started?*

Guest: Yes.

Salesperson: *In spite of the initiation fee isn't the real issue one of value? That is knowing that the value you will get from your program here will far outweigh the initiation fee? I mean, if six months from now you were getting all the things you wanted from a program, wouldn't it have been worth it?*

Guest: Maybe, I guess.

Salesperson: *Well, John, how much more then you expected is the initiation fee?*

Guest: I really had not thought there would be an initiation fee at all, but I would think collecting the first month's dues would be reasonable.

Salesperson: *John, I know you want to feel better about yourself and be healthy and I know that you are concerned about the initiation fee; but isn't your health more important than $150.00?*

Selling Fitness

I WANT TO CHECK OUT OTHER CLUBS

Salesperson: *You want to check out other clubs?*

Guest: Yes, I want to check out all my options.

Salesperson: *That's fine, I can appreciate the fact that you want to check out all of your options. If you don't mind me asking, is there something in particular that you are looking for that you did not find here?* (Of course, his answer to this should be, "No" because on the way back to the sales area you already asked him a question which pre-handled this objection.)

It is my personal opinion that unless you really close hard with him, a guest using this objection is going to check out other clubs. For whatever reason, he is not convinced that your club is the place for him. If nine times out of ten he will leave no matter how hard you close, let him leave-but preframe him on what to look for. In order to do this, you must know everything you possibly can about your competition.

You want to give your guest a brief overview of the other clubs, pointing out the pros and the cons of each in respect to the guest's needs and wants. One rule though, is <u>never bash the competition</u>. Be professionally honest. If you know that another club has something that the prospect wants and your club does not have it, tell them. If you know one of the programs they have is not as suited to his wants as your program, tell him that as well. If you know that a club has a policy of hard closing, drop him a hint to be prepared for a different type of presentation and to not be bullied into a membership. In the long run he will respect your honesty. **Remember, with no discernible difference in products, you make the difference!** The conversation might continue something like this:

Guest: No, your club is fine, as I mentioned though, I just want to check out all my options.

Closing & Overcoming Objections

Salesperson: *I can respect that. Although you may want to visit all the clubs in the area, from what you have told me, I think you can safely narrow your choices down to three clubs; A club, B club and ours. The reason I say that is C is a Gym, with free weights only. Since the aerobics program is of most importance to you, some of the things you will want to evaluate are availability, variety of classes, size of the studio, certification of instructors and flooring.*

I know that both A & B clubs have early morning classes and unless they have changed their schedules in the last month, I'm pretty sure that we are the only club with a late evening class. As far as cost is concerned, I know that both clubs monthly dues are a little less than ours, but I think that when you tour the clubs and weigh out all factors, you will understand why our dues are ten dollars more a month.

Lastly, John, I cannot stress enough the importance of you feeling totally comfortable with the people and the environment of the club you choose. It will do you no good to join a club that you don't enjoy going to. I know that only you can know what environment is best for you. At the same time, I would be remiss if I did not forewarn you that you may feel a bit more pressured to buy at some of the other clubs. Until someone actually visits other clubs they do not realize how different our way of doing business is.

<u>If your club truly is better than your competitors, you shouldn't have to worry about the guest going to look at other clubs</u>. If you pre-frame him as to what to look for he may come back sooner than you think, appreciating your honesty.

If your club has a "first visitor discount" that you are strict with, (and, by the way, that is the only way in which it will really work), you may want to try and get the guest to put the membership on hold before they leave the club. The conversation might go something like this:

Selling Fitness

Salesperson: *John, I completely understand your wanting to check out other clubs. Let me ask you, if there was a way that you could take advantage of your first-visitor discount and go check out other clubs, would you be interested in that?* (I have seen very few guests who are serious about joining say, "No" to this question.)

Guest: How could I do that?

Salesperson: *If you would like, I can ask my manager if you could put the membership on hold. If he approves we would go ahead and fill out all the paperwork; you could leave a small, fully refundable deposit and then go check out the other clubs. If you decided that this club was for you, you would still get the savings. If you decided to enroll somewhere else you could just stop by and get you deposit. Would you like me to ask him/her?*

A "hold" is a great option that many people will take you up on. <u>The most important part of the "hold" technique is putting the final decision on the manager's shoulders</u>. You don't want the guest to think that you have the authority to offer the hold because that will make the option less credible.

I'M NOT SURE I AM GOING TO STICK WITH IT

Salesperson: *You're not sure you are going to stick with it?*

Guest: That's right.

Salesperson: *John, I'm sure you have reasons for saying that, do you mind if I ask what they are?*

Guest: As I mentioned before, I joined a club and then after two months I stopped going.

Closing & Overcoming Objections

Salesperson: *So, if it weren't for the fact that you quit before, in your opinion would you get started?*

Guest: Probably.

Salesperson: *Probably or yes?*

Guest: Yes, I think I would do it.

Salesperson: *Well, if that's the case, let me ask you a question. Let's suppose that you and a friend decide to come to the club. You are on a free trial membership and your friend pays full price to get started. Suppose that both of you get busy with work. Which one of you will be more committed to maintaining an exercise program during that period, the one who made the financial commitment or the one who paid nothing?*

Guest: Well, of course, the one who made the commitment.

Salesperson: *(Go right to the close) John, if that's the case isn't that the very reason you should just make the commitment now?*

I NEED TO TALK TO MY SPOUSE

Salesperson: *You need to talk to your spouse?*

Guest: Yes, I never make a big decision like this without talking with her first.

Salesperson: *I can understand that. John, just out of curiosity, what do you think she will say?*

Guest: I'm sure she won't have a problem with it.

Salesperson: *It's just a common courtesy thing that you want to discuss it with her?*

Selling Fitness

Guest: Yes.

Salesperson: *Just suppose for a moment that you were not married. If that were the case, would you go ahead and get started today?*

Guest: Yes, probably.

At this point you have two options. You can close again by saying:

Then why don't we go ahead and fill out all the paper work and you can call me with the final okay.

Your second and less aggressive option, would be:

Great, what I would suggest then is that we set up a time for your first workout with the fitness staff. At that time we will complete all the necessary paperwork. What day is better for you, Thursday or Friday?

Of course, I could spend hours writing out sample scenarios for overcoming each common objection. Every sale is unique! Therefore, your conversation with each guest is going to be slightly different. However, the core questions that get to the heart of the objections (as scripted out in this chapter) must be woven into each conversation. Also remember, the best way to handle objections is to pre-handle them so that you don't have to overcome them at the close. If, though, you have mastered the basic steps for overcoming objections and are sincere about helping others, you will soon find yourself easily dealing with objections and making lots of sales.

Closing & Overcoming Objections

SUMMARY

1. Once you and the prospect are finished with the tour and are sitting down ready to go over the memberships, you want to ask him one final question: "Aside from membership affordability, do you have any other questions?"

2. Even if you know that the guest's needs and wants fit perfectly into one of your memberships, show them all of the memberships. Of course, spend more time going over the features and benefits of the program that best suits their needs and just skim over the others pointing out why it is not a good choice for them.

3. Once you ask for the sale, be quiet!

4. Welcome objections. They give you an opportunity to solve a problem and close the sale.

5. Once a guest gives you an objection, nicely feed it back to him. Next, align with him; question it; isolate the objection; reframe it, and; finally, close again.

6. If the guest does not purchase a membership that day, it is very important that you establish a course of contact with him.

EXERCISE

The only way that you are going to get comfortable with overcoming objections is to memorize the steps outlined in this chapter, and then practice applying and using them with the most common objections in live, role-play situations.

1. Memorize the basic steps for overcoming objections.

2. Practice presenting your membership options to co-workers and have them give you one of the more difficult common objections. Stay "in" the role-play and try to overcome their objections. Have the language given to you in this chapter memorized and then begin to customize your statements to the situation at hand.

10

THE POWER OF PROSPECTING

As a sales trainer I am constantly being told by salespeople, "You know Casey, I have a great closing ratio once I get someone in the door, but I just can't seem to get enough people in front of me." Anytime I hear that, I know the salesperson hasn't yet caught onto the concept of prospecting.

All too often salespeople are so caught up with struggling to make this month's numbers that they haven't had time to stop and figure out that if they prospected, they wouldn't be struggling! Once someone actually sits down and calculates-numerically-the benefits, they will never look at prospecting in the same way. So, right now I want you to take out your calculator and do the exercise below.

2	3	5
x 2	x 3	x 5
x 2	x 3	x 5
x 2	x 3	x 5
x 2	x 3	x 5

What does all this multiplication mean? Well, if two people knew about your product or service and they told two, who each told another two people, and if that happened just four times, you would end up with a total of 32 people hearing about your product or service.

Selling Fitness

Next, if you start out with 3 people who tell three people, and so forth, you end up with a whopping 243! Stop and look at those two final figures. There is a big difference between 32 and 243. The most fascinating thing about these two numbers is that although the difference in their totals at the bottom is 211, the difference in their beginning numbers is just 1! Meaning that it takes just one more person at each stage to produce 211 more individuals who know about you and your product or service.

And just to show you how incredible the exponential growth of prospecting is, I had you do the same thing with 5. As you have figured out, you end up with 3,125! Even if you think it is unrealistic that members would tell five people, (they will if you are giving them incredible service) cut the number in half. I would take 1,062 knowing about me and my product or service any day of the week!

STRENGTH IN NUMBERS

Can you see the incredible power in these numbers? Just think of how many people you come in contact with, both inside and outside the club! The potential you have for prospecting and the financial rewards you will reap from it are limitless. So, how do you tap into the power of prospecting? The first step is understanding the difference between prospecting and networking. Let me do this by way of analogy.

A fisherman places his nets into the ocean, scoops up everything he can and then pulls the nets onto the deck of the boat. Once the nets have been emptied he begins to pick through the fish that he has caught, looking for only those fish that are the right type and size which can be sold on the market. Therefore, in order to get one box of fish, he might have to pick through quite a few nets of fish.

The Power of Prospecting

As the salesperson, you are going to cast your net out via networking. That is, you are going to let as many people as possible know about your product or service. Once you have pulled your net of prospects in, you are going to pick through them, searching for those people that have the correct amount of interest and desire to purchase a membership. The focusing of your efforts on qualified individuals is prospecting. <u>The entire process is simply a numbers game. The bigger your net, the more fish you will catch</u>!

To sum up that analogy, networking is the process by which you try and let the masses know about you and the club. Prospecting is when you are actively contacting and pursuing an individual who had shown some interest in enrolling.

TAKING THE RESPONSIBILITY

Although there is no disputing the fact that if you let more people know about your products and services you're going to make more sales; many salespeople seem to be confused as to who is responsible for letting potential prospects know about their products and services. Too many salespeople think that it is the club's job to generate leads-but it is not!

If, when training new salespeople, there was just one thing that I could teach them, it would be that they are responsible for their own sales. Let us use the fishing boat analogy again. If your club is the boat, and the owner or manager is the captain, that makes you one of the crew members. When the fishing boat goes out to sea and is ready to cast the nets out, it's not the boat or the captain who does that-it's the crew. You see, the boat (or club in your case) is just the vehicle which allows the nets to be effectively cast, and the captain (that's the owner and manager) is up in the wheel house steering so that you don't get off course.

CAST YOUR NETS!

As a salesperson, you have to put your own nets out to generate your own prospects. If you aren't generating a majority of business for yourself, and most of your sales come from walk-ins and telephone inquiries, you're not a professional salesperson. You are more like a retail salesperson selling only to those who walk into your store with a certain level of interest already.

I must tell you though, in all of my years in this business, I have seen very few people who have established a solid networking and prospecting system. For many years, fitness salespeople didn't have to network because money was plentiful. Clubs could afford to spend a bundle on advertising, and people were just walking in the door and signing up. Well, you and I both know that those days are over. Today, competition is fierce and clubs have to operate a lot leaner. That means that you-as a professional salesperson-will have to network and prospect. So, where do you begin? The backbone of creating a good network is having a solid in-club referral program.

THE BEST KEPT SECRET

When asked, "What is the best source of leads available," ninety-five percent of salespeople answer, "Referrals." Why then, do less than just twenty-five percent of salespeople consistently ask for referrals? One probable reason is that many clubs do not have a referral policy or system to follow. More accurately, though, what prevents salespeople from tapping into the rich resources of referrals is fear of rejection. Not only are salespeople afraid of being told, "No, I don't want to give you any names," but many feel that although the guest has agreed to buy, they do not want to do anything which would make the guest back out of the sale or come back to cancel.

The result is the salesperson neglecting to ask the new member for names and numbers at the point of sale. "Maybe later, after I have serviced him for a while," he thinks. Well, if you have given one

The Power of Prospecting

hundred percent of yourself to the guest and truly care about him, he will want to give you names and numbers.

Now, some of you may be saying, "What's the big deal? I don't consistently ask for referrals but it obviously doesn't hurt my sales-I make my quota every month." My reply is, "There are only two ways you can increase your productivity, work harder or smarter." With the already demanding hours of the health and fitness industry, I would choose working smarter over harder any day of the week. Having a good referral program is like owning a franchise. You have people all over the place working to generate income for you, and you don't even have to be present! Remember our multiplication chart? When you obtain referrals you are multiplying the number of potential pre-qualified prospects you have to work with at an incredible rate. What is even better, is that with referrals, someone else is doing most of the groundwork for you! Basically there are two types of in-club referrals; point of sale and existing member. Before we get into the specifics of each, let's talk very generally about how to set up a referral system.

HAVING THE PASSES

As simple as it may seem, the first step to having a productive referral program is having passes. Believe it or not, not all clubs have an actual guest pass. Some clubs use their business cards with "guest pass" written on it. This is not acceptable, particularly for new member referrals. Not having guest passes is like a traveling salesperson not having a brochure on the product he represents. Today's consumer is very educated and having some makeshift promotional material will not cut it. **Remember that a guest pass is a reflection of you and your club, make sure it projects the image you want to create.**

Although it is not necessary, I recommend that you have two different passes: seven-day and one-day. Aside from just not asking, one of the biggest reasons salespeople do not get a lot of buddy referrals

(BR's) from new members is that they do not give value to passes. You need to present the passes as something specially done exclusively for new members. <u>One way to do this is by giving only new members seven-day guest passes. In addition, put a limit on the number they are eligible to receive. Make sure that the one-day passes are given out at all other times.</u> The only exception to this rule should be a one-time special occasion that centers around an annual event, making it the only time of year where seven-day passes are given out to any member. Be prepared though, if you have been handing out seven-day passes at free will, your old members will fight this at first. They have been spoiled. If you stick to the new system; they too will grow to appreciate and respect those special occasions where seven-day passes are given out. The end result will be an increased percentage of the passes getting used because they have value.

THE FORMAT

The passes do not have to be elaborate, but a few pieces of information are crucial. First, the club's phone number. Second, spaces to fill in the member's name and the guest's name. Next is a place for an expiration date. This is important because you want to create a sense of urgency to use the pass. Remember a guest pass is a tool for you to create business in the immediate future.

```
               One Week Guest Pass
    Name: _____
    Guest of:  _____
    Exp. Date:  _____
    Consultant:  _____
    Offer available to first time guests, age 18 or older.
         By appointment only:  Call 401-792-7009
```

To see sample guest passes, please visit www.MarketMyClub.com

The Power of Prospecting

Last and most importantly, the pass should be clearly noted "**by appointment only**." Unless it is perfectly clear that the pass can be used by appointment only, what is a potential sale could turn into a nightmare.

Imagine that you are in the middle of a great tour with a guest and one of your members walks in with a buddy referral wanting to talk to you about enrollment. One of a few things could happen. First, you could make an attempt at working with both guests, juggling them between locker rooms, machines, and desks, which will probably result in a major loss of rapport. Let's face it, people know when they are being juggled and, unless they are extremely sheltered, they know that you work on some sort of commission. What will probably run through their mind is, "If this is the way I am being treated before I have paid my money, how will I be treated afterwards?"

A second option is to have the guest sign a waiver of release, to work out with his friend this time, and schedule another time to come in and work with you. This is no good either because you are not in control of the guest's visit. His friend could give him misinformation, work him out too hard, too easy. And, any number of things could go wrong. In addition, if that guest eventually becomes a member, a bad precedent has been set.

A third choice would be allowing the guest to work with another salesperson. The problem with this option is that the very elements that make a BR such a quality lead; pre-established rapport, trust, and reciprocity, are no longer present with another salesperson. The bottom line is that if you can prevent it, you do not want referrals to unexpectedly visit the club. Make sure "By Appointment Only" is clearly seen on all passes. Also, reiterate the policy to the new member, so that when he gives the pass to his friend he will tell him to call first.

BUDDY REFFERAL FORM

<u>The next element of a quality referral program is having some type of form for the new member to fill out</u>. The form must look professional and explain how the system at your club works. This is extremely important. I know of so many clubs that spend a lot of money having very nice guest passes printed, but were not getting the number of referrals they should have because they skipped on the BR form. The form is the vehicle for social proof. It sends the message that this is your policy. Americans are conditioned to believe that what is in print is truthful. Don't use a scrap piece of paper or a writing tablet. As simple as it sounds, this is a must. On the next page is an example of a simple, yet very effective BR form.

WHEN TO BR?

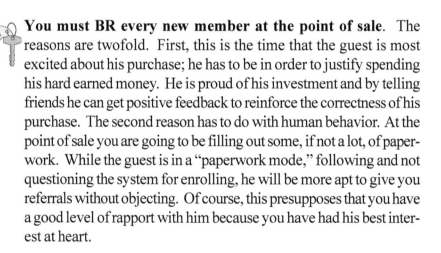

You must BR every new member at the point of sale. The reasons are twofold. First, this is the time that the guest is most excited about his purchase; he has to be in order to justify spending his hard earned money. He is proud of his investment and by telling friends he can get positive feedback to reinforce the correctness of his purchase. The second reason has to do with human behavior. At the point of sale you are going to be filling out some, if not a lot, of paperwork. While the guest is in a "paperwork mode," following and not questioning the system for enrolling, he will be more apt to give you referrals without objecting. Of course, this presupposes that you have a good level of rapport with him because you have had his best interest at heart.

The Power of Prospecting

NEW MEMBER GUEST PRIVILEGES

Dear New Member,

Congratulation on your decision to begin an exercise program here at ABC Club.

One of the privileges of becoming a new member is that at the time of enrollment you can receive up to five one-week guest passes, allowing five different friends of yours who live locally to use the facility free of charge for an entire week. That is a $_____ value!

Please fill out the form below to register your friends.

Member Name:_____
Date:_____ Membership#:_____
Home #:_____ Work #:_____

WHO COMES TO MIND?
*Family   *Friends   *People you socialize with
*Neighbors   *Co-Workers   *Friends who work out

        Name: Phone#:

1. _____   _____
2. _____   _____
3. _____   _____
4. _____   _____
5. _____   _____

Selling Fitness

THE PRESENTATION

Once you have closed the sale and you are getting ready to do the paper work, that is the time to BR. You should be saying something along these lines:

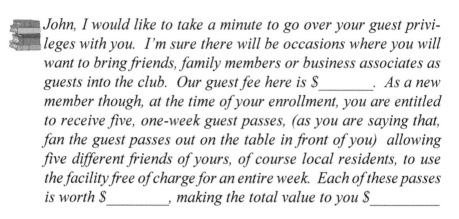

John, I would like to take a minute to go over your guest privileges with you. I'm sure there will be occasions where you will want to bring friends, family members or business associates as guests into the club. Our guest fee here is $_____. As a new member though, at the time of your enrollment, you are entitled to receive five, one-week guest passes, (as you are saying that, fan the guest passes out on the table in front of you) allowing five different friends of yours, of course local residents, to use the facility free of charge for an entire week. Each of these passes is worth $_____, making the total value to you $_____

While I am completing your paper work, I need you to fill out this form with the names and contact numbers of those people you want to register to receive one of these passes.

Now, place the BR form and a pen in front of him, gesturing for him to begin filling it out. **Do not wait until you are done with the paperwork.** Having him work on the form while you are doing the paperwork accomplishes two things. First, it gives him something to do and keeps his mind on something other than the mound of paperwork, which can be intimidating to some people. Second, it gives him time to sit and think of as many names and phone numbers as possible. If you have taken the time to get to know him, established a good level of rapport, have let him know verbally and non-verbally that you want to make a difference in the quality of his life, the majority of people will give you some names.

Although many salespeople think the job ends here; you are not finished yet. It is absolutely imperative that before your new member leaves the club, you get information about each and every one of his referrals. What is his relationship with that person? Are they exercising now? If so, what? Have they exercised in the past? Have they ever been a member of a club before? Why does this person think they will be interested in using the pass? general fitness, weight loss? How does that person feel about themselves right now? Are they married, single? Where do they live in relation to the club? You have got to do your homework so that when you call the referral you feel as if you already know them and can more easily establish rapport with them.

DEALING WITH OBJECTIONS

Even when you have a great relationship with the customer, there will be some people who will be reluctant to give you names and/or phone numbers. Let's discuss some of the objections you will hear.

"I can't think of anybody right now."

This objection is probably the most common one you will hear. As was the case with the "I need to think about it" buyer's objection, the "I can't think of anybody right now" referral objection is usually the result of the member being afraid that you are going to call up his friends and pester them about buying a membership. The first thing you want to do is to try a simple re-direct. One long-time club manager successfully uses this statement:

John, let me ask you, what was the biggest purchase you have made in the past year or so? (Whatever they say, a car, a stereo, new furniture, you go on to ask them this:) *Well, who was the first person you showed it to? The second person?*

Continue this until he cannot think of any more names. If he still cannot (or will not) give you any names, don't get upset. Let him know that he will have the opportunity to use them at a later date:

Selling Fitness

That's fine, what I will do is place your buddy referral form in your file and when you can think of those people that you wish to receive the passes, you can come and see me. You have sixty days to use your one-week passes. After that I can only give you one day passes.

By doing this you are accomplishing a few things. First, you are creating a reason for keeping in touch with him. Second, you are giving value to the passes. You are conveying the idea that these passes are special enough to need a registration slip. In essence, you are saying to the new member, "We are going to keep track of these because you only get a certain number." Lastly, having a system like this taps into the law of scarcity. If the member comes to you to get another pass and you say, "Let me check to see if you have any left and if they are still eligible," his brain will place value on the remaining passes. Maybe he will be more selective of the friends he gives the remaining passes to, choosing those that are the most serious.

Creating value, using the law of scarcity and establishing a relationship that requires ongoing contact are the three elements you want present when dealing with all objections regarding BRing. Here are two other common objections, and the statements you can use which will keep you in the driver's seat.

"Can I take this paper home and bring it back?"

At one time, I never let a member take home their buddy referral form. The reason being "Out of sight, out of mind" for both the salesperson and the member. They would take the paper home and it would get lost somewhere, and the salesperson would soon forget that the member had not given him any names. I have since found a way to let the member take a sheet home without allowing those potential referrals to fall through the cracks. Therefore, when a member asks you if they can take the form home, your reply should be this:

The Power of Prospecting

Because the club keeps track of all of these guest passes, I have to turn a form in with your other paperwork. If you would like, I'll put this one in your file and will give you an extra one to take home and bring back."

Make sure that they fill out the top part of the form and finish up by telling them to turn the form into you when they come into the club next time, as well as nicely informing them when the passes expire.

"Why don't you just give me the passes and I will fill them out when I decide who I want to give them to?"

To this question you have a very easy and justifiable response-the passes have a dollar value and can't be floating around without a name and the proper authorization. Your response to this question might be something like this:

Because these are 7-day passes, we can not just hand out blank ones. I'll tell you what I can do; I can give you the guest passes of those people you know that you want to give one to. I will then file your registration form so that in the future, when you think of someone else, I can register them and give you the pass.

In some cases, a new member will give you names, but is reluctant to give you the phone numbers of his friends. <u>When this happens, on option is to ask the member for the buddy's address so you can send the pass along with a note.</u> Sending a pass to a referral by mail may spark interest, or at least make the buddy feel somewhat obligated to use the pass now that is has been sent.

As long as you are committed to helping people enjoy the benefits of a regular exercise program, you should feel comfortable asking for phone numbers and addresses. Remember, most people think about getting started on some sort of fitness program, but they need to be motivated to take the first step. Further, you have collected enough information from the new member giving you the

Selling Fitness

reasons why this person may be interested in using the club. It is your job to do whatever it takes to get them to give fitness a fair chance.

WHEN TO CONTACT NEW BR'S

How quickly do you want to follow up on the new member BR's? <u>You should be making the initial attempt at contact within the first week</u>. Studies have shown that you have about a thirty day window to get referrals into the club. You want to get the buddy into the club while your new member is still excited about the club and enthusiastic about wanting his friends to join with him. Below is a script that you can use for making BR calls. As you will see, it is very similar to the info call.

THE BR CALL

Hi, is (Name) there?

(Name), you don't know me yet, but a friend of yours, _____,referred me to you, how are you today? The reason for my call is that_____ is a new member here at the ABC Club, has he/she told you yet? Well, _____ was given a certain number of special ____ week guest passes to give to friends and family and he/she has chosen you as one of the recipients! My name is _____ and _____ told me that you......(feed back to him some of the information you got from the new member regarding his fitness needs and wants), *is that so?*

(Now you move into the probing stage of the info call. Use present or past tense language depending on whether they are working out or not.)

- ☛ *What type of activity was it/is it?*
- ☛ *How long ago?*
- ☛ *How many times a week?*
- ☛ *How long did/have you stick/stuck with the program?*

The Power of Prospecting

- ☞ Did you/are you getting the results you want/ed?
- ☞ If so, why did you stop?
- ☞ Or what aren't you getting that you want?
- ☞ Finally, have you noticed any difference in how you feel?

If you don't mind my asking, what specifically would you like to accomplish with a health club membership?

(Name), That's great because we have _____ here.

What I would like to suggest, and I think you would agree, is that the best way for you to find out if the club is going to help you reach your goals, is that we set you up for a time to come in and begin using your free pass, how does that sound?

What hours will you be using the club, morning, afternoon or evening?

I have an opening this _____ or _____, which is best for you?

(Name), do you know how to get to the club?

When you get to the club check in with the front desk and let them know you have an appointment with me, again, my name is _____. (Slight pause) The visit will probably take around _____, so plan accordingly. (Tell them about workout clothes, etc.) (Slight pause)

Someone from the club will be giving you a courtesy call the night before just to confirm and I ask only that if for some reason you are unable to make your appointment please give me a call as soon as possible because I work by appointment only, okay?

I look forward to working with you on _____ at _____, have a nice day.

Selling Fitness

SHOULD I CLOSE?

Many people ask me, "When someone comes into the club with a seven day guest pass should I try to close them on the first visit?" One really can't say definitely yes or no to this question-it all depends. It goes back to the test closes we talked about in the tour procedure. You have got to find out where your guest is in his decision making process. By all means, if he is ready to be presented, show him the memberships. Maybe he has been thinking about this for months and is ready to buy. But, if the guest is not really responsive to your test closes throughout the tour and workout, then don't try and close him. Give him the space and respect he deserves. Remember you want to build a level of rapport with the guest, where as even if he doesn't become a member of the club, he will give you a good reference.

Some clubs have printed right on their guest pass that if redeemed on the first visit the pass is worth a certain amount off the membership. This too has pros and cons. For the guest who is almost ready to buy, this might be enough of an incentive. For the guest who is serious about considering a membership, but needs the week to try it out, sometimes he gets angry at the fact that he has been given the week then penalized for not enrolling on his first visit. He does not appreciate "sales tactics" which try to pressure him into signing on the dotted line so quickly.

When deciding whether to try and "close" a BR on his first visit, keep in mind that it is a proven fact that one unsatisfied guest will tell more people about his negative experience with a salesperson or a facility than a satisfied person will. Don't get a reputation for being obnoxious or pushy; in the long run it's not worth the few sales you will be able to close.

EXISTING MEMBER REFERRALS

The key to obtaining lots of existing member referrals is positive relationships. The bottom line is, if members like you, they will give you referrals. One way to maintain positive relationships with

The Power of Prospecting

members is by staying in contact with them, and I'm not just referring to saying "Hi" to them when they are at the club. **The professional salesperson keeps in contact with his members over the phone.** All too often, the only time a member hears from a salesperson via phone is when their membership is up for renewal.

I encourage all salespeople to contact all of their members on a rotating schedule-even if it's only once every few months. The first time you call a member, don't be surprised if they ask you "Is everything alright," "What do you want," or "Am I late with my payment or something." When you say, "No, everything is fine, I just called to say hi, how are you, how are your workouts going or is there anything I can do for you," after they get over the shock, they are very grateful that you cared enough to take the time to call them.

Although contacting your members by phone is a very important part of obtaining referrals, you never want to ask for referrals when doing these phone calls. In addition, make sure you don't ask them for names the very next time you see them in the club. If you do either of these things, it will look as though the only reason you called them was to set the stage for asking for referrals.

Besides being a very professional and courteous business practice, making phone calls to your members pays off in the long run. Remember, when you get to know your members not only is it easier to approach them about referrals, but once they like and trust you, they begin to come to you when they have someone who is interested in membership.

TRACKING EXISTING MEMBER BR'S

It is important that you have a system for tracking buddy referrals after your new member has used their original seven-day passes. Many times as a manager, I would have fitness counselors come up to me and say, "Casey, I gave out twenty passes today, isn't

Selling Fitness

that great?" My response was, "That's nice. Great is when you have the twenty names and phone numbers to go along with them!" (Refer to the guest pass register illustrated below.)

When you give out a one-day pass, write down the name and phone number of the member you are giving it to. If he will give you the name and or number of his guest, get it. Also, note the expiration date you placed on the pass. This gives you a great reason to follow up. As the date approaches call up the member and ask him who he gave the pass to. Remind him when the expiration date is and that it can be used by appointment only. Finally, if he doesn't know when he and his guest will be coming in, try and get him to tentatively set a date. Ask him to call you if he and his guest cannot make the appointment. Of course, all of this tracking can be done with computers.

GUEST PASS TRACKING FORM

Date	Mbr's Name	Phone #'s	Guest	Phone #'s	Exp.	F/U

EVEN A SIMPLE FORM WILL ALLOW YOU TO
KEEP TRACK OF GUEST PASSES GIVEN OUT

CREATIVELY GENERATING LEADS

Although generating leads from within the club is the most logical and simple type of prospecting, top salespeople in any industry create a much broader base of business for themselves. One of the reasons a salesperson needs to have a good mix of referral sources is that different promotions bring in different types of people. Therefore, when one source of prospecting is not working, a salesperson isn't left with a limited number of prospects to work with. Your prospecting outside of the club will fall into different categories: personal prospecting and promotional prospecting.

PERSONAL PROSPECTING

Personal prospecting is just as it sounds-prospects you get from your own individual efforts. Although the number of prospecting ideas that you create and implement is solely up to you, here are a few successful ones.

COMMUNITY NEWSPAPERS

As simple as it sounds, there is a ton of leads in your local community newspaper. Any announcement, whether it be a graduation, marriage, or a new baby, is a potential prospect.

What you do is cut out the announcement and send it to the person. Along with the clipping you send a letter. If it's to a newlywed the letter should discuss the importance of regular exercise to health, stress release and maybe something on the benefits of doing social activities with your spouse, particularly when that activity is a healthy one. If it's a new mom, the letter should discuss the importance of post-partum health care and, if your club has any class that is geared to moms and their babies, send some information on that. If your club has day care, discuss the benefits of having that service to make exercising easier for her, both logistically and mentally. Of course, with every letter you put a one-week guest

Selling Fitness

pass to the club with an expiration date on it and a note that says "First visit by appointment only."

When someone receives a newspaper clipping on themselves it is like getting a gift and that person will be thankful that you took the time to send it. Even if they don't use the pass, you are getting out in the community in a positive way.

SERVICE INDUSTRY

Another great source of leads is setting up a referral program with other professionals in a service industry. For instance your hairdresser. Hairdressers are perfect because they are talking to people all day long-people who are concerned about how they look. You can set up a program with your hairdresser where she gives out passes to her customers with her name on them. If you can work it out that she gets their permission to forward you their name and phone number, all the better for you. When a person calls or visits the club because of her guest pass, give her a free week of membership. If they enroll, give her a free month. If that amount of time seems too generous, adjust it to be a fair reflection of the value that has been given to you.

Of course, with hairdressers and other service industry people (tailors, dry cleaners, manicurist, massage therapists, etc.) you can set the arrangement up on a continual basis. That is, they continue to get membership to your club, while they are still actively giving out guest passes. The reason I don't like this arrangement is that they don't have as much incentive to get people to actually walk through the club doors and enroll. A happy medium to these two scenarios would be to place a lead box in their store and membership would be contingent upon the box producing leads.

When thinking about setting up referral programs with other businesses or independent service people, keep in mind that, just like any "sale" you need to be able to show them what is in it for them. If they might be a great source of leads but they are not interested in

The Power of Prospecting

membership for themselves, are there any creative options available to you. For instance, if it is a business that has many employees, could he use the membership time in smaller pass increments, offering them to employees as an incentive or bonus program. Whatever you do, make sure that the program is a win-win situation or else they will not want to do it.

COMMUNITY SPEAKING ENGAGEMENTS

<u>If you are the type of person who doesn't mind getting up in front of small or large groups; companies and organizations love to have people come in with health and community awareness programs-particularly when they are for free!</u> While working at one club, every year we went and spoke to groups of IBM secretaries at a special dinner the company had for them. In addition to talking to them about the many benefits of exercise we did a short demonstration on the different styles of aerobics classes we offered and then left them all with one week guest passes into the club as well as a coupon for a free body fat analysis. The employees loved it because they were getting something of value and the company loved it because it made them look good. We loved it because we ended up with over one hundred prospects to work with.

PERSONAL CONTACT

Very early one morning, I was on my way to give a seminar and I stopped at a Dunkin' Donuts to get a cup of tea. A man was in front of me in the line, paid for his coffee and donut and left. About a minute later he appeared again, handed me his business card and said, "My name is _____ and I'm the most successful Better Homes real estate agent in this county. I noticed you were from out of state. If you or someone you know is looking to move into this area, please give me a call. I will do whatever I can to help you. Have a nice day," and he left. Now, I have to tell you, although I didn't keep his card (because I had no need for a house in that area) the man left me with a great impression. You can bet that if I was interested in a house-or even knew of someone who was-I would have considered

Selling Fitness

giving him my business. Anyone who is passing cards out to total strangers at Dunkin' Donuts at 5:30 in the morning probably is the most successful real estate agent around. I would want a go-getter like that to be representing me in finding a home.

The same concept holds true for you as a professional in the health and fitness industry. <u>If you pro-actively and professionally introduce yourself to people, and let them know with confidence and energy that you help people get more enjoyment out of life by involving them in a regular exercise program, I guarantee you that a certain percentage of people will show an interest.</u> They might strike up a conversation with you, call you, come into the club or even pass your card along to someone who does have an interest.

The bottom line is that every single person that you come in contact with outside of the club should know exactly how you might be able to help them, or someone they care about, by way of an exercise program at your club. Although some new salespeople are reluctant to tell people (particularly strangers) about what they do, as a professional you should feel confident about your products and services.

PROMOTIONAL PROSPECTING

The difference between personal prospecting and promotional prospecting is really the size of the project. Personal prospecting is usually on a smaller scale and generates an amount of leads that a salesperson can handle themselves. On the other hand, promotional prospecting is done on a large scale and usually involves all of the other salespeople at the club. Although many salespeople wait for the club to design and organize promotions, top salespeople are pro-active at planning promotions throughout the year in an effort to maximize their own income. Of course, the benefit of a larger promotion is that it can create a much greater level of excitement among the staff, existing members and potential prospects. Again, there are hundreds of different promotions that can be run. Here are just a few ideas to get you thinking.

CAR DEALERSHIPS

There have been many clubs that successfully run promotions with car dealerships. Often, what the dealership does is give the club a one-year lease on an automobile to be used in a referral contest. For every new guest that a member brings into the club, the member gets a raffle ticket to put in the bin. If their guest enrolls, the member will get five raffle tickets. Therefore, the more people the member introduces to the club, the greater their chances are of winning. This provides a great source of leads for every salesperson.

As far as the dealership is concerned, in addition to having the club put up posters and flyers promoting them, very often they will actually bring the car to the club and prominently display it in the parking lot or by the street (of course with signage). This gives them additional advertising to people other than members. The promotion can be run anywhere from two to four months and will produce hundreds of leads.

T-SHIRT GIVE-AWAY

Another great referral program is the "Preferred Member Program." This program works particularly well in the summer when traffic is traditionally slower. It does have an initial expense, but generates hundreds of names. Have T-shirts with your club logo printed on them. Underneath the logo, have the words "Preferred Member." The shirts should be good cotton shirts, nicely done, and visually attractive. Next, go back to your computer and generate a form which has "preferred member" written at the top and underneath that have spaces for ten names and phone numbers of friends, with a brief description of how the program works. That is, when a member gives you the names and number of ten friends who would like a free visit into the club, even if the people decide not to come in, the member gets the T-shirt.

Selling Fitness

I don't know what it is about T-shirts, but everyone wants them, especially if they are nice looking. In addition to having signs about "Free T-shirts. Ask me how" all over the club, the salespeople go onto the fitness floor with a T-shirt over one shoulder and a clip board with the preferred member forms in the other. They will ask members, "Did you hear about our preferred member program?" When the member says, "No," the salesperson proceeds to tell them that the club is giving away great T-shirts (As that is being said they hold the T-shirt up for them to see) to any member who gives the name and contact numbers of five people who they think might be interested in coming in for a free fitness evaluation and workout at the club. They should reiterate to the member that there is no obligation to them. They will get the T-shirt just for referring the individuals, even if they decide not to come into the club. Of course, the salesperson then asks, "Does that sound like something you would be interested in?"

If you are wondering why we have only asked the member for five names when the form says that ten names must be given, it is just a way to make the member feel more confident that they can come up with five names. If they see the "form" with ten names but you only ask them for five, they are more likely to think, "Hey, some poor guy had to give ten names for the shirt but I'm only being asked to give 5, I can do that."

If you and your club have a good reputation of not being pushy, this promotion will generate a lot of names. In addition, if you only print a limited number of T-shirts, ensuring that you run out of them before everyone earns one. This way when you run the promotion the following year, people will act faster.

FUND RAISERS

<u>Although I can't credit it as being my own idea, a great fundraising idea is to have local athletic groups or organizations sell very short term (like a week or two) memberships</u>. They sell for a very nominal amount, maybe five or ten dollars. The member-

ship forms are done on small, numbered, 3x5 NCR forms which captures all the necessary contact information. One copy of the form goes to the purchaser, one goes to the organization and one comes back to you at the club. The purchaser gets a wonderful trial membership, the organization gets to keep the money and you get the prospects to work with, as well as some great PR in the community. In addition, I think it is a lot better seeing some of these youth organizations sell fitness passes instead of candy bars, but perhaps that is a little bit of a biased opinion!

As you might imagine, the possibilities for prospecting and networking are endless, and only limited by your imagination and willingness to try something different.

SUMMARY

1. Referrals are the most powerful source of lead generation. In addition, referrals are the best quality leads to have.

2. The guest passes your club has made are extremely important to the success of a referral program. The passes do not have to be elaborate, but having certain information on the pass is crucial: The club's phone number; spaces to fill in the member's and guest's name; a place to write-in an expiration date, and; having "By appointment only" printed in a place where it will be seen by everyone.

3. Always BR at the point of sale, and have a professional looking BR form that the member fills out at that time.

4. Remember, you want to give the passes value; use the law of scarcity and create a reason to keep in touch.

5. Make the first contact with buddy referrals within a week after getting the name.

6. If on their first visit, a BR gives you a good indication that he is ready to buy, present the membership and ask for the sale. If, however, he does not appear ready to buy, do not risk losing rapport with him by presenting the memberships. Instead, keep in touch with him, talking with him after each of his visits and measuring his level of interest.

SUMMARY (cont.)

7. Once a new member has taken advantage of his 7-day guest passes, you will want to continue getting referrals from him. Do not just give out one-day passes, make sure that you are tracking who you give them to, who the guest will be and the expiration date you placed on the pass.

8. In addition to buddy referrals, top salespeople look for many other ways to build a solid base of leads to work from. Personal prospecting and promotional prospecting can help you build your business.

9. Some personal prospecting ideas include reading the community newspaper for announcements, forming referral programs with people in a service business, speaking at community or business events as well as pro-actively handing out business cards.

10. Some promotional prospecting ideas include programs with car dealerships, T-shirt give-aways and fund raisers.

11. Remember the possibilities for prospecting and networking are endless. Be willing to use your imagination and try something different.

EXERCISE

1. Memorize the New Member BR presentation and then practice it with co-workers.

2. No matter what, give every new member the BR presentation.

3. During your first few weeks on the job, make it your business to introduce yourself to every member that you can. Keep a BR tracking form with you at all times and, as you start to recognize faces, ask people if they have any friends who would like to come into the club for a free visit. Approach them from the standpoint that you are new and would like to work with as many people as possible.

4. Aside from people you know, what places do you frequent that might be ideal for setting up a referral program with? List them out.

5. What other places of business in your community might prove to be good "business partners" for a referral program? List them out.

11

LEAD MANAGEMENT

Although it is not the most exciting to discuss, lead management is a very important part of successful salesmanship. The fact is, having an effective lead management system results in an increase in your sales productivity regardless of your natural ability to sell.

Interestingly enough, when consulting with clubs, both big and small, I frequently find that they have no lead management system. In fact, what I often find is that their "system" is a folder full of old needs analysis sheets mixed in with a million little slips of memo notes that have names, phone numbers and comments written on them. One may wonder why a lead management system is so instrumental in helping a salesperson produce more than his average, unorganized counterpart.

WHY LEAD MANAGEMENT?

The first reason is that a lead management system is efficient. When a salesperson keeps all his leads piled in one folder, he has no systematic way of knowing who he should be calling on a particular day or in a particular month. In July he may come across a lead that says, "Call back in April." Calling a prospect back three months after the fact will look very unprofessional. In addition, if a salesperson does not have his leads organized, potential prospects will fall through the cracks, resulting in his making fewer sales and experiencing a greater amount of frustration.

Selling Fitness

Therefore, it only makes sense that salespeople who have an efficient lead management system are less apt to experience fluctuations in the number of memberships they sell each month. <u>Because they know exactly who to call and when to call, they close a greater number of prospects who might have never bought if the salesperson not been persistent with their follow-up.</u> As a result, during traditionally slower selling periods, salespeople who have lead tracking systems will maintain a higher degree of success.

Another very important reason for having a lead management system is that, in the fitness business, there really is no such thing as a dead lead. Just because someone has an interest in fitness and walks into your club, it doesn't mean that they are ready to join right away. Maybe they will decide to start with a home exercise program or will join a community program. Maybe they will leave and do nothing about their level of fitness at present. That does not mean, though, that at some point in time in the future they won't be ready to get started. If you keep in touch with prospects, not to nag or bother them, but just to check in with them and find out where they are in terms of their commitment to making a lifestyle change for the better, they will be more apt to buy from you when they are ready.

Even a guest who visited your club and decided to join somewhere else is still a potential future prospect. Their membership is going to eventually run out. If they are not happy with the place they are at, they will be a prime candidate for enrolling at your club, particularly if you keep in touch with them, even if it is only via e-mail.

<u>What most salespeople don't think about is that if you have implemented an effective lead management system, you can create powerful lists.</u> With the use of computers, you can radically increase the effectiveness of your clubs advertising dollars by targeting select direct mailing pieces and/or e-mail campaigns to previous guests. In addition to being more effective than traditional advertising, the beauty of direct mail is that it costs a lot less. Instead of the club having to

take out a very expensive ad in a newspaper that may or may not be seen by an individual who is interested in a membership, your direct mail pieces go out to people that you know have an interest in what you offer. <u>An added benefit of direct mail is that by keeping in touch with prospects that didn't even buy anything from you, you are creating a reputation as someone who cares</u>. This helps you and your club to build long-term relationships with the people of your community. That, in and of itself, is priceless.

Aside from keeping in touch with prospects so that you will sell more memberships, another reason why you should have a good lead tracking and management system is that the statistics you can derive from your tracking are great diagnostic tools. Such statistics will tell you exactly what you need to work on in your quest to become a better salesperson. How successful are you at getting info-callers to set appointments? What is the show ratio for your info callers? And what is your membership closing ratio? These are just a few of the statistics that will indicate to you what you need to work on.

Perhaps the most obvious and often discussed reason for good lead tracking is the fact that, in an effort to make the phones ring, your club spends thousands of dollars on different types of advertising. That allows you to sell more memberships. If you want management to spend their money intelligently, and in a way that is going to best support you, they need to know objectively and quantifiably what is working and what isn't. The only way that you can do that is by providing them with accurate information that will come from quality lead management.

THE CHALLENGE

As you can see, the benefits of a good lead tracking system are many. By implementing any type of system, you will greatly enhance your level of success and your income. The challenge, though, is getting salespeople to begin using a lead tracking system. The fact is that organizational skills are something that many, many salespeople have difficulty with. Most salespeople do not enjoy dealing with details, particularly paperwork or other administrative tasks.

Add to this the fact that the most valuable thing to a salesperson is their time. If you are not in front of prospects touring them or on the phone trying to set future appointments, you are not maximizing your time. As a result, salespeople have a hard time justifying spending the time to set up a lead management system.

Another reason that implementing a lead management system can be difficult is the fact that it isn't something that is absolutely necessary to being successful. Unlike many traditional sales positions where the salespeople go out and generate almost all their own leads and contracts, fitness salespeople are in the fortunate position of having many prospects delivered right to their door via telephone inquires or walk-ins. Because of the steady stream of leads, some fitness salespeople can be relatively successful without even keeping in touch with past prospects. As a result, not having to really work leads creates an environment of complacency and salespeople can get accustomed to what I call "Gimmee" sales. The professional fitness salesperson, though, follows a prospect's buying cycle for six, twelve, twenty four or more months, keeping in touch with them until they are ready to buy.

AUTHOR'S NOTE

Please keep in mind that the first printing of this book was in 1994, before computers were a standard piece of equipment in clubs. Today, some 18 years later, most salespeople have a computer at their workstation. That said, instead of completely deleting the "archaic" parts of this chapter, I have kept them because I believe the fundamental concepts are still applicable. Further, as crazy as it seems to some (particularly those under the age of 30), there is still a place for old fashioned organization of some papers you use at the club. In particular, you will have many Needs Analysis forms from previous guests. You will never input all of their personal information into your

Lead Management

lead tracking system. Therefore, many salespeople will keep these forms and refer back to them during the follow up process.

So, as you read the remainder of this chapter, give some respect and appreciation to the computer sitting at your desk.

SETTING UP THE SYSTEM

The good news about a lead tracking system is that getting started is easy and doesn't require any major expense. Probably the simplest way of organizing leads is by using a hanging folder system. Whether you have a desk file drawer or you invest in a portable file box, it doesn't really matter. Many people also use the same basic system with a large index box. That is okay, but it adds an unnecessary step. Instead of being able to file needs analysis sheets directly into a hanging folder, you will have to transfer the prospect's information onto an index card.

Label your file folders from 1-31 and January through December. That will give you a total of 43 files. Obviously, the file folders numbered 1-31 are representative of the days of the month. If you know you need to follow up with a prospect on a particular day, you will file their card or information in the appropriate file. That way, when you get into work, you pull out the folder for the day and know exactly whom you need to call or write to. You use the month files when someone wants you to get back to them in a time period that is greater than a month. So, if it's August and a prospect tells you to call them back in three months then you would put them in the file folder marked November and when November comes around you pull out the file and place the leads in the appropriate 1-31 folders.

IT'S EASY TO USE!

It's a pretty straightforward system but let's work through a scenario to see how the lead will move from file to file. When an incoming phone call comes in, you immediately begin recording the

Selling Fitness

information they give you down on your club's telephone inquiry sheet. You do a good job at probing and staying in control, get all the necessary information and you close them on an appointment for coming in on the 19th of the month. On the back of the inquiry sheet or in a space that is designated for follow-up notes, write the date of the appointment down. After you log the appointment into your appointment book, you immediately go to your file system and put the telephone inquiry sheet into the folder that is numbered 19.

When you get into work on the 19th of the month, you pull out the folder for that day and your scheduled appointment will be there. Suppose the appointment shows up, they are toured and presented memberships, but they do not buy. You set a follow-up date of one week, which would make that the 26th. After they leave the club, you would make the appropriate notes on the needs analysis form, then file the form in the folder marked the 26th.

Now, what if when you call the prospect on the 26th day they tell you they need two more weeks to make a decision because they're going on vacation. Where would you file their card then? Your first reaction might be to put them in the next months file folder, but that wouldn't be the most efficient place to put it. <u>As long as the date you need to follow up with someone is less than 30 days from the present day, you are always going to put them in the appropriate 1-31 day files</u>. Now, as simple as that sounds, for some reason that gets people confused. So, let me give you an illustration. If today is the 15th of January, your file folders from the 15th to the 31st will represent the rest of January, but the file folders 1-14 will represent the leads for the first two weeks of February. Therefore, with our example, if we talk to the prospect on the 26th of the month and they tell us to call them in two weeks, their card is going to go into the appropriate day folder, 7th, 9th, or 10th. That will depend on the number of days in the present month.

Next, let's suppose you call the prospect back in two weeks and they tell you they aren't ready to make the commitment. Instead of just hanging up the phone empty handed, you will want to get their permission to check in with them in two or three months.

Lead Management

Again, not to nag or bother them about buying, but to find out how they are doing in terms of their fitness goals. Of course, you would note the conversation and then put their card in the appropriate month's file. Now, there comes a point where a lead becomes very cold and, instead of continuing to follow up with phone calls, you may want to put them on a mailing list. This will be more productive for your time and less threatening to the prospect-but they still need to be kept in contact with.

ENHANCING THE SYSTEM

When I was selling memberships full time, in addition to the file folders discussed, I also had an additional set of file folders for every month that was labeled "Mailers." After I had spoken to a prospect a few times on the phone, I transferred their card to the "Mailer" files and kept in touch with them via note cards and flyers, as discussed in the chapter "Making the Most of the Telephone." Of course, today most of this follow up will be done via e-mail but the concept still applies.

<u>Another thing that you can do to further enhance your lead management system is to sort by category of interest</u>. Within each month of mailer files you may want to separate the leads by the primary concern of fitness, or that area of the club that the prospect was most interested in; weight loss, mature market, kids programming, aerobics, etc. Then, if and when your club runs a special membership, which is very suited for that particular area, you can quickly and easily pull those leads and target your mailer accordingly. It goes without saying that if you have access to a computer and you stay on top of entering leads, the amount of time it will take to put out mailings is significantly reduced.

DO IT NOW!

So, the system is pretty straightforward and basic, but the bottom line is that it works. Where many salespeople get into trouble is moving from the "I need to do this stage" to the "I've done this stage." All too often, salespeople will go out and get their folders, set

Selling Fitness

them up but then don't start using them because they think they need to first get all their old leads organized. <u>That's not necessary!</u> The best thing that you can do is set up your folders and start organizing you new leads-today-right now. Then, as you start to plow into the piles on your desk, file them accordingly. Don't try and fight your time constraints, work with them. Much to your surprise, in a couple of weeks you will have disseminated and filed all the leads that had piled, and in the process, you will probably have uncovered a number of prospects that had fallen through the cracks!

KEEP ACCURATE NOTES

<u>Although it should go without saying, the final point I wanted to make about this system is that your notes on contact dates and what transpired are crucial to the success of your follow-up</u>. I don't care how good your memory is. If you are touring 5-10 guests a day and contacting and following up with another 20-30 prospects a day; there is no way in the world you are going to remember when you last spoke to someone, what was said and the course of action that was decided upon. You have got to get into the habit of writing notes down and I'm not talking about lengthy writings. Codes are fine: SI for still interested. CB 4/99 for call back in April of 1999. LM for left message. NA for not available. NI for not interested. The important thing is that your system be verifiable and your codes understandable so, at a glance, you know what the situation is and what needs to happen next.

Although I am not at your club forcing you to set up a lead management system, I highly encourage you to make the commitment to doing so. I can guarantee you that if you force yourself to get into the habit of using the system, the rewards will far outweigh the effort. Just as those people new to a fitness program come back and tell you how much better they feel physically as a result of their new membership, after sticking with your lead tracking system for a month of two, you will look back and say "How did I ever live without it."

SUMMARY

1. Having an effective lead management system results in an increase in your sales productivity regardless or your natural sales ability.

2. One reason a lead management system is so important is because it creates efficiency, allowing you to know whom to call and when. This prevents leads from falling through the cracks.

3. Another reason lead management is important, is that there really is no such thing as a dead lead in the fitness industry. Fitness is something that can be started at any time in one's life and is continuous. Even if a guest becomes a member at another club, that does not mean that they won't consider your club some day.

4. Having an effective lead management system allows you to create powerful mailing lists, and to direct promotions to those individuals that are most receptive to the offer.

5. Also, the statistics you can track from your lead management system can be used as a diagnostic tool for how you are doing at each stage of the selling process.

6. Because your club spends thousands of dollars to make the phone ring so you can sell memberships, you need to accurately track where your leads are coming from. An effective lead management system allows you to do this.

7. The challenge that many salespeople have with lead management is getting themselves to use it. Often, a lack of organizational skills coupled with time constraints is enough to push salespeople into procrastination mode with a lead management system.

SUMMARY (Cont.)

8. Getting started with a lead management system is easy and does not require any big expense. File folders and a drawer or box to hang them in is all that is necessary.

9. A very important part of a lead management system is noting all the conversations you have had with a prospect as well as future contact dates. By creating a coding system, note taking will be much easier.

EXERCISE

1. Take a look at your clubs current lead management system. If they have one, how efficient is it? Write out the pros and the cons.

2. If your club does not have a lead management system, go out and purchase a portable file-folder box and get your file system set up. Begin filing all your new leads immediately and gradually work through and file older leads as you go.

CONCLUSION

So, we have come full circle in the selling process, covering everything from the pre-sale to the post-sale. I know that I have given you a lot of information-much more than can be mastered in one reading. Therefore, in order to integrate the material and get the most out of this book; I recommend that you keep a copy of Selling Fitness close at hand, re-reading chapters and referring to sections as the need arises. Repetition is the mother of skill! Whether you are a brand new salesperson, experienced, but new to the industry, or are a veteran, I hope that Selling Fitness has provided you with materials that make your job of selling health club memberships easier and more enjoyable. I would like to leave you by sharing a poem that my grandmother taught me.

Be the Best of Whatever you Are

If you can't be a pine on the top of the hill,
Be a scrub in the valley but be
The best little scrub by the side of the hill;
Be a bush if you cant be a tree.
If you cant be a bush be a bit of the grass,
And highway happier make;
If you cant be a muskee then just be a bass-
But the liveliest bass in the lake!
We can't all be captains, we've got to be crew,
There's something for all of us here,
There's big work to do and there's lesser to do,
And the task you must do is the near.
If you cant be a highway then be a trail,
If you cant be the sun be a star.
It isn't by size that you win or you fail-
Be the best of whatever you are!*

-Douglas Malloch

*Best Loved Poems of The American People. Garden City Books of NY, 1936

Made in the
USA
Middletown, DE